CW01083131

A handb

For Elsevier Butterworth-Heinemann

Publishing Director: Caroline Makepeace
Development Editor: Kim Benson
Production Manager: Anne Dickie
Design Direction: George Ajayi

LASIK

A handbook for optometrists

Michelle Hanratty BScHons MCOptom

Refractive Clinic Manager, Aston Academy of Life Sciences,
Birmingham, UK

Foreword by

Emanuel Rosen BSc MD FRCSE FRCOphth FRPS MAE

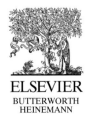

ELSEVIER
BUTTERWORTH
HEINEMANN

EDINBURGH LONDON NEW YORK OXFORD PHILADELPHIA ST LOUIS SYDNEY TORONTO 2005

ELSEVIER
BUTTERWORTH
HEINEMANN

ISBN 0 7506 8809 2

British Library Cataloguing in Publication Data
A catlogue record of this book is available from the British Library.

Library of Congress Cataloging in Publication Data
A catalog record for this book is available from the Library of Congress.

Note
Knowledge and best practice in this field are constantly changing. As new research and experience broaden our knowledge, changes in practice, treatment and drug therapy may become necessary or appropriate. Readers are advised to check the most current information provided (i) on procedures featured or (ii) by the manufacturer of each product to be administered, to verify the recommended dose or formula, the method and duration of administration, and contra-indications. It is the responsibility of the practitioner, relying on their own experience and knowledge of the patient, to make diagnoses, to determine dosages and the best treatment for each individual patient, and to take all appropriate safety precautions. To the fullest extent of the law, neither the publisher nor the editors assumes any liability for any injury and/or damage.

The Publisher

 your source for books,
journals and multimedia
in the health sciences
www.elsevierhealth.com

The
Publisher's
policy is to use
**paper manufactured
from sustainable forests**

Printed in China

Contents

Foreword

Eye care in the 21st century is a team affair. The interdependence of optometrist and ophthalmologist in the UK sets an example to the rest of the world where competition rather than co-operation is the norm.

The ametropic patient now has options. Do they wear spectacles, which are usual during childhood and adolescence, or do they graduate to contact lens wear? Once mature, however, a permanent correction for ametropia becomes a reality in our new world of refractive surgery, which is the fastest growing sub-speciality in the field of ophthalmic surgery. It takes many forms which include corneal laser surgery, providing the bulk of the possible treatments, and also utilises lenticular options through phakic lens implantations and refractive lens exchange. The indications for each potential application include the degree and type of refractive error, the age of the patient (presbyopia is a major issue), the physical dimensions of the eye and within the eye as well as the visual needs and expectations of the patient. I emphasise the distinction between eye and patient. It is so easy to concentrate efforts on an eye and its refraction before and after treatment, but it is the outcome for the patient which is all important. Ocular dominance, mild amblyopia, binocular function, near, intermediate and distance vision are all contributors to the decision making equation facing the refractive surgeon. The risks and benefits of interventions, sensible patient expectations and ability to cope with setbacks, however infrequently they may occur in the surgical population as a whole, are issues and potential burdens that the eye care team have to acknowledge.

Geography plays a role also and makes shared care so important, which returns to the theme of a team concept for patient service and management. The optometrist's role is to recognise the indications for surgery as well as its happy outcomes and occasional complications. Patients' needs include the imparting of sensible and considered advice based on continuing education and awareness of what is possible whilst leaving the surgeon to finally advise the patient on what is appropriate for them as well as a consideration of risks and benefits. Too often in the past patients have received inadequate or inappropriate counselling to their detriment and, in the end, that of the advising optometrist. That is why this volume when carefully read and absorbed should help to avoid the pitfalls in the management of patient counselling both pre-operation and postoperation. It should help to avoid alarmist comments for patients tend to dwell on professional advice as though it is the last word which of course it is until they receive the specialist's opinion. The point is that once ideas enter the heads of some patients they are hard to be dissuaded of the notion even though it may be incorrect.

Continuing professional development, progressive education, advancement of knowledge, appraisal, revalidation, litigation, malpractice; just some words that describe the burden of modern professional life. Thus any written contribution that eases those burdens is most welcome. I am sure this volume will be appreciated by the optometric profession and am honoured to be invited to introduce it.

Emanuel Rosen BSc MD FRCSE FRCOphth FRPS MAE
Visiting Professor, Department of Optometry and Vision Sciences at the University of Manchester Institute of Science and Technology. Director Rosen Eye Clinic, Co-editor *Journal of Cataract & Refractive Surgery.*

Preface

Optometry is now a diverse profession and many optometrists are becoming involved with shared care schemes in both the private and public sector. Although there are certified training courses for some glaucoma and diabetic schemes within the NHS, it is up to individual laser refractive surgery providers to ensure that appointed optometrists are adequately trained to co-manage their patients.

The aim of this book is to complement any existing training by providing a comprehensive guide and on-going reference source for optometrists who are working within the field of laser refractive surgery. It will also provide some insight for optometrists not involved in any co-management schemes, but who want to learn more about laser *in situ* keratomileusis (LASIK).

The optometrist's role throughout the patient journey is described in detail with chapters dedicated to the interpretation of clinical data, patient management and postoperative care. A typical treatment procedure is also included for those who want to provide more information about the procedure to patients who are interested in having LASIK. Refractive surgery is a continuously evolving field with new techniques emerging that may eventually supercede existing ones. The final chapter discusses whether the surface ablation technique laser epithelial keratomileusis (LASEK) will become the treatment of choice in the future.

Used in routine practice, this handbook will enable optometrists to discuss laser refractive surgery so that the patient can be better informed about all possible options for vision correction. In co-management, the handbook will serve as a reference tool to ensure that patients continue to receive appropriate postoperative care from the co-managing optometrist.

Michelle Hanratty

Dedication

This book is dedicated to my family, friends and colleagues for their encouragement and support while writing this book.

Acknowledgements

I would like to extend my warmest thanks to Emanuel Rosen for writing the foreword to this book, and also to thank Wayne Crewe-Brown and Mark Wevill for checking clinical content, William Harvey, Frank Eperjesi, Andrew and Ngaire Franklin for advice on specific chapters and to Shehzad Naroo for general feedback.

Chapter **1**

Guidelines, regulations and standards

OVERVIEW

This chapter outlines the regulations and guidance that an optometrist working in the refractive surgery field should be aware of. It takes into consideration the guidance from the Royal College of Ophthalmologists and the College of Optometrists and discusses the General Optical Council regulations. The Association of Optometrists has also released an advice document for its members and the details are incorporated into this chapter. Details of the Healthcare Commission regulatory role are also included. The acceptance of refractive surgery in various occupations varies from one occupation to the next. This chapter will enable the optometrist to advise patients that are interested in joining those occupations which have high visual standards.

CONTENTS

INTRODUCTION

The public demand for laser *in situ* keratomileusis (LASIK) and alternative forms of refractive surgery has risen exponentially over the last few years. The UK is following the trend set by the US where laser eye surgery is seen as almost commonplace. Increasingly, patients are considering laser eye surgery as an alternative way of correcting their ammetropia, with contact lens wearers twice more likely to consider surgery than spectacle wearers.[1]

The market has responded to this trend with more clinics opening.[2] Skilled ophthalmologists are in demand and, ultimately, their time is best managed if optometrists share the pre- and postoperative care of patients. While some optometrists are actively working in specialised clinics, more and more optometrists are using refractive surgery as a way of both growing their practice, and increasing their involvement in primary eye care.[2] Despite wide optometric participation in patient co-management schemes and in refractive surgery clinics, there is very little peer guidance on the optometrist's role, responsibility and liability in this environment.

SHARED CARE SCHEMES

The concept of shared care is now well established with many hospitals using optometrists in programmes which monitor conditions such as primary open angle glaucoma and diabetes. The Royal College of Ophthalmologists has issued some guidelines with respect to shared care within the Hospital Eye Service[3] and which could also be used as a basis for good quality shared care schemes with private clinics. The guidelines which were produced in consultation with The Royal College of General Practitioners and The College of Optometrists cover many aspects ranging from the set-up of schemes to the training of non-qualified staff.

The guidelines state that the participation of such schemes must be based on individuals rather than practice based, and that protocols relating to the scheme should be agreed beforehand by all the participants. The protocols 'should clearly define who has clinical responsibility at any one time and what those responsibilities are'. They should also state who has overall clinical responsibility and specify the functions to be carried out by each participant. On-going training is required to ensure that the participants understand the management strategies for this shared care scheme. There should also be a method of rigorous review of the scheme to ensure that it remains effective.

The Association of Optometrists (AOP) has also produced a resource pack for the setting up of shared care schemes in primary eye care.[4] This is a particularly useful guide if the optometrist is planning a local arrangement with a surgeon who does not currently have an established protocol for the co-management of patients. It gives examples of existing schemes as well as details of how to create a shared care framework and how to establish protocols.

The College of Optometrists currently has guidelines which relate to photorefractive keratectomy (PRK) but not to LASIK.[5] More inclusive guidelines with respect to all forms of refractive surgery have yet to be produced. In these guidelines, there is some reference to co-management of patients postoperatively. It is the duty of the optometrist to ensure that they possess the knowledge, skill and instrumentation to carry out the required clinical examinations. The guidelines also state that it is the optometrist's responsibility to ensure that they have undertaken the necessary additional training to participate in such schemes. The view is also stated that the clinical responsibility of the patient should always remain with the ophthalmologist that carries the treatment.

The General Optical Council (GOC) statement on PRK[6] dates back to March 1995. New guidelines are currently being produced but, at the time of writing, these had not yet been published. Existing guidelines are specific to PRK and as such do not encompass the more recent treatments such as LASIK. The policy is clear in stating that clinical advice, counselling and aftercare relating to PRK is only carried out by optometrists that have received adequate training in accordance with the guidelines set out by The College of Optometrists. The policy also covers rules relating to contractual agreements with excimer laser clinics and the payment of fees. This latter issue will be discussed later.

CONTRACTUAL AGREEMENTS AND CO-MANAGEMENT FEES

This refers to partnerships or contracts between refractive surgery clinics and optometric practices. The College of Optometrists Advice to Fellows and Members – PRK[5] was published in January 1995 and consists of two sections. The first deals with route of referral and optometrist training, the second deals with the ethical implications of entering into agreements with excimer laser clinics. The guidelines indicate that the optometrist should ensure that the clinics to which they refer provide treatment to an appropriate standard and that they themselves do not enter into any agreement which may compromise their professional and clinical freedom. It advises that any link between the referring practitioner and the treating clinic must be on a purely professional basis. Accepting fees or other inducements for referring patients for treatment is considered highly unethical and is not acceptable practice. Referral of patients must be based solely upon clinical judgement and not subject to pecuniary influences.

The *Standards for Photorefractive Surgery* document was published in December 2003 by The Royal College of Ophthalmologists[7] and gives more specific guidelines for co-management and other issues. In section 5 on clinical governance, it states that incentives should not be offered to professionals in return for the referral of patients for refractive surgery.

The GOC statement on PRK (1995)[6] is very clear on its position and states that fees or other inducements for referring a patient to a particular clinic should not be accepted. The GOC accepts that fees can be paid for work undertaken including advice prior to referral and for postoperative care. It indicates that work prior to treatment should be paid for by the patient and that postoperative care can be paid for by the treating clinic. The arrangements should be made clear to the patient 'at the outset to avoid the risk of bias or unethical behaviour'. It also states that the GOC has accepted the guidelines issued by The College of

Optometrists as peer view and that any breach of these may constitute serious professional misconduct.

The co-management schemes that are currently set up between optometrists and clinics usually involve the optometrist carrying out some pre-operative assessments, giving advice to the patient about treatment, and then postoperative care in their own practice. In return for these services, the clinic pays the optometrist a fee. This is not a referral fee but a co-management fee. It could be argued that the fees paid for the co-management chair time is far greater than the charge for the equivalent number of eye examinations. This is true. Therefore, does this amount to an incentive to refer for treatment? On the other hand, it is also true that the average private eye examination fee is not representative of the real value of the qualification, knowledge, and instrumentation required to perform that examination and that the resultant spectacles dispensed would compensate for this. Therefore, it could be argued that a reasonable co-management fee should be equivalent to the expected income generated from the sale of spectacles, not just the chair time itself.

THE CONSENT PROCESS

If carrying out pre-operative assessment, the optometrist needs to be aware of the guidance issued on the consent process by The Royal College of Ophthalmologists in the *Standards for Photorefractive Surgery* document.[7] If a patient wishes to pursue treatment, they must receive a consent document to read at least 24 hours prior to surgery so that they have enough time to read and understand the information. The person carrying out the pre-operative assessment is responsible for ensuring that any questions arising from the consent form are addressed and that the patient fully understands the treatment expectations, potential complications and other treatment options. The patient should also have an initial consultation with the treating surgeon at least 24 hours before treatment. This is to rule out any unsuitable patients and so that the surgeon can ascertain that the patient has fully understood the risks and benefits of treatment.

Other published information that should also be made available to the patient at the time of initial consultation includes:

- the treatment(s) available at that clinic and the eligibility criteria for patients
- the risks and benefits of each treatment
- statistical information regarding the visual outcomes and complications
- the professional qualifications and experience of the surgeon.

POSTOPERATIVE CARE

After the patient has had treatment, the first aftercare is usually carried out by the ophthalmologist at the clinic. Further routine aftercares are usually carried out by an optometrist either in a clinic or in their own practice if part of a co-management scheme. It is The Royal College of Ophthalmologists' view that the surgeon is responsible for ensuring that postoperative care is carried out appropriately.[7] It is also the optometrist's duty to ensure they have undergone the appropriate training,[5] and that they are only carrying out procedures that have been agreed in the co-management scheme protocol.

While co-managing a refractive surgery patient, the optometrist should only carry out procedures or make clinical decisions for which they are qualified and trained. Where the patient presents with a postoperative problem the optometrist must decide whether or not the management of that condition falls within their remit.

Management of dry eye

The rules relating to injury or disease of the eye (1999)[8] permits optometrists to manage ocular conditions without referring to a GP if it is in the patient's best interests. The optometrist can manage dry eye with the use of ocular lubricants and punctual occlusion. Some ocular lubricants can be found on general sale in non-pharmaceutical outlets and are often found among contact lens products, *e.g.* Refresh. These can also be supplied by the optometrist. Other ocular lubricants such as hypromellose and Viscotears are pharmacy medicines and as such can only be supplied via a signed order to a pharmacist unless in an emergency.

The College of Optometrists has also issued specific guidelines for the use of punctum plugs.[9] Optometrists must ensure that they have the required knowledge about the clinical application of puntum plugs and their possible sequelae. The guidelines also give the following advice:

- a full clinical history should be taken and the symptoms indicating the need for punctal occlusion noted
- diagnostic tests that are carried out to confirm that puntum plugs are needed should be documented
- written information about the procedure and the follow-up regimen should also be given to the patient
- informed consent should be obtained in writing and kept with the patient's record card
- optometrists need to ensure that patients are informed about the source of collagen-based products and to follow correct sterilisation procedures to prevent cross-infection
- the patient's GP should be kept informed about any advice given or procedures carried out.

Further information regarding the control of cross infection can be found in the *Cross Infection Control in Optometric Practice* booklet from The College of Optometrists.

Management of ocular infection

The optometrist is only able to manage eye conditions with specific topical agents which are:

- listed in schedule 5 of The Prescription Only Medicines (Human use) Order (1997)[10]
- on the General Sales List
- classed as pharmacy medicines.

The Royal Pharmaceutical Society (RPS) publication *Medicines, Ethics and Practice: A Guide for Pharmacists*[11] states: 'ophthalmic opticians may sell or supply certain medicinal products provided it is in the course of their professional practice and in an emergency'. If the situation is not an emergency, the medicine can be supplied by a pharmacist where 'the sale or supply shall be subject to the presentation of an order signed by a registered ophthalmic optician'. Therefore, if a patient presents with signs or symptoms of a microbial infection and the optometrist feels referral back to the treating surgeon is unnecessary, a signed order for an agent such as chloramphenicol may to written. These guidelines can be viewed on the RPS website <www.rpsgb.org.uk> in the members section under 'law and ethics'.

DEALING WITH AN EMERGENCY

The optometrist is given some general guidance from The College of Optometrists regarding the management of ocular emergencies in routine practice.[12]

- if the optometrist conducts an emergency eye examination, it should be made clear to the patient that only the presenting symptoms are being addressed and that a routine eye examination is still required in due course

- if the optometrist does not examine the patient's eyes, referral to an appropriate healthcare professional is required; the patient should be informed of the degree of urgency

- if the patient contacts the practice by telephone only, the optometrist should advise the patient to come into the practice or seek alternative medical attention; all advice should be recorded.

In the shared care of refractive surgery patients, protocols should state the appropriate procedure in an emergency. For example, if an optometrist is working in a clinic without a surgeon in attendance, and a patient presents with signs of late onset diffuse lamellar keratitis, what is the appropriate course of action? If diagnosed, the treatment for this condition would normally be a steroidal agent prescribed for topical use with the frequency depending upon severity of the condition. Regulations prevent the optometrist from supplying or prescribing a steroidal agent even in an emergency as they are classed as prescription only medicines. The appropriate course of action would be to refer the patient to the treating surgeon urgently. If this was not possible, then urgent referral to the GP or to a hospital eye department with arrangements to see the surgeon at the next available opportunity is necessary.

In some cases, the surgeon may be happy to confer with the optometrist over the telephone and decide upon a temporary management regimen until the patient can be seen. If a prescription is necessary, it would need to be sent directly to the pharmacy. In such cases, the surgeon is relying on the observations of the optometrist but the legal responsibility of prescribing remains with the doctor who signs the prescription.[13]

LEGAL PROTECTION

The AOP has issued advice in its handbook relating to optometrists and co-management of refractive surgery patients[14] which can be divided into three main areas:

- **Contract** – a written contract of employment or for services should be drawn up which includes details of the tasks or procedures that the optometrist is required to carry out. It should also indicate that the ophthalmologist under-taking treatment accepts responsibility for all advice and procedures that have been delegated for that patient.

- **Advice to patients** – the optometrist is able to inform the patient about differ-ent treatments, but should not advise the patient to have treatment. The patient could pursue a claim for negligence against any professional advisor in the event of an unsuccessful outcome. It is therefore important that the optometrist only advises on procedures that they themselves are undertaking. The final decision for suitability and specific advice regarding surgery should be given by the sur-geon. The patient should also be advised if the optometrist has any co-management arrangements with the clinic they are being referred to.

- **Professional indemnity insurance** – AOP professional indemnity insurance will provide cover for any work that might be normally undertaken by an optometrist, including pre and post-operative assessments. It will not cover for procedures or tasks which an optometrist is not qualified to carry out. The AOP also advises that the optometrist should ensure that the clinic or ophthalmologist that they are working with is insured against claims made by patients and that this indemnity insurance will cover the optometrist during the period of contact for any claims arising out of advice or work carried out, and for any future claims.

COMMISSION FOR HEALTHCARE AUDIT AND INSPECTION (CHAI)

On 1st April 2004, the roles of several commissions were brought together to form the CHAI and is also known as the Healthcare Commission. The new national body was established by the Health and Social Care (Community Health and Standards) Act 2003 and took over the role of regulating and inspecting the independant healthcare sector which had previously been carried out by the National Care Standards Commission.

Independent health care – national minimum standards regulations

These are a set of minimum standards that are published by the Secretary of State for Health in accordance with the *Care Standards Act (2000)* which must be adhered to by clinics to gain and retain registration with the CHAI.[15] Essentially they require the clinic to provide: (i) patient-centred services thus ensuring patient safety and quality assurance; and (ii) clear and accurate information for patients.

The manager of the clinic is registered with the CHAI and is accountable for the compliance of the clinic to these minimum standards. There are eight core standards:

- information provision
- quality of treatment and care
- management and personnel
- complaints management
- premises, facilities and equipment
- risk management procedures
- records and information management
- research.

These standards are comprehensive and cover the fundamental principles such as taking informed consent, to the minutiae of wearing name badges. There are several standards that relate to professional staff and can be referred to on the Department of Health website <www.dh.gov.uk> in the Policies and Guidance section under National Care Standards Commission.

OCCUPATIONAL REGULATIONS AND REFRACTIVE SURGERY

There are some occupations which restrict entry into service for those who have undergone refractive surgery. There is no blanket rule to cover all occupations or all refractive procedures. Regulations are constantly under review and are subject to change. Up-to-date information is available from the AOP members handbook[16] in which amendments are issued as required or from various government websites.

The Royal Navy

Candidates applying for entry into the Royal Navy that have undergone refractive surgery of any type are not currently accepted. Serving personnel who have had refractive surgery are medically assessed to determine their fitness for duty. Personnel are also informed that the surgery 'could well have an adverse affect on their future career by rendering them unfit for duty, due to potential side effects'.

The Army

The Army will accept candidates that have undergone some forms of refractive surgery only. Each case is judged individually by the Army Medical Board after an examination. Applicants that have had radial keratotomy (RK) or astigmatic keratotomy (AK), or intraocular surgical procedures are not accepted. Those candidates who have had LASIK, PRK or intrastomal corneal ring segments (ICRS) may be accepted if they can also provide documentary evidence to fulfil the following criteria:

- the pre-operative refractive error was not more than ±6.00 dioptres spherical equivalent in either eye
- the best corrected acuity is 6/6 or better in the right eye and 6/12 or better in the left eye
- 12 months or more must have elapsed since the date of the last surgical procedure
- there must be no significant visual side effects secondary to the surgery that affects daily activities
- refraction must be stable as defined by two refractions carried out at least 6 months apart, with no more than 0.50 dioptres difference in the spherical equivalent in each eye.

The Royal Air Force

Prospective applicants that have had refractive surgery will not be accepted for aircrew or specialist branches. If the candidate is recommended as suitable for entry by a Service-approved consultant ophthalmic surgeon, then acceptance into non-specialist ground branches is permitted. The candidate is also required to produce documentary evidence to support that:

- the pre-operative refractive error was not more than +8.00 or −7.00 dioptres along the highest powered meridian in either eye
- 12 months or more must have elapsed since the date of the last surgical procedure
- refraction must be stable as defined by two refractions carried out at least 6 months apart, with no more than 0.50 dioptres difference in the spherical equivalent in each eye.

Pilots

Joint Aviation Requirements (JAR) are issued by the Joint Aviation Authorities which can be divided into two classes. Class 1 relates to commercial pilots and airline transport pilots. Class 2 relates to private pilots only. After refractive surgery, a class 1 pilot is grounded for a minimum period of 1 year following surgery. An assessment with a Civil Aviation Authority ophthalmologist is required 6 months and 12 months postoperatively. A medical certificate can be issued at this second assessment if the following criteria are met:

- the pre-operative refractive error was less than ±5.00 dioptres along the highest powered meridian, and no more than 2.00 dioptres of astigmatism
- satisfactory stability of refraction

- no increase in glare sensitivity
- postoperative refraction and vision must be within the appropriate JAR limits.

Class 2 pilots have the same conditions apply after treatment, except that a medical certificate can be issued after a 6 month assessment with a local ophthalmologist if the JAR criteria are met.

Air traffic control officers and other personnel

Air traffic control officers, flight engineers and flight navigators are also subject to regulations issued by the Civil Aviation Authority. After RK or PRK, the applicant is grounded for a minimum of 1 year following surgery. An assessment with a Civil Aviation Authority ophthalmologist is required 6 months and 12 months postoperatively.

Police

The latest vision standards and acceptability of applicants who have had refractive surgery can be found from the Home Office website www.homeoffice.gov.uk.[17] Applicants who have undergone RK, AK or corneal grafts will be rejected due to the side effects of these treatments. PRK, LASIK, Laser epithelial keratomileusis (LASEK), ICRS and epi-flap procedures are acceptable for recruitment provided that:

- a minimum period of 6 weeks has elapsed following treatment
- there are no residual side effects
- all other requirements of the vision standard are met.

Applicants may be asked for documentary evidence regarding their eyesight. The eyesight form that needs to be filled in by the optometrist can be downloaded from the Home Office website.

Fire service

The current guidelines were issued in a Fire Service Circular issued by the Home Office in 1996[18] are new guidelines are under review. Although some brigades specify that they do not accept any surgical eye correction, this may change in the near future. Some brigades do accept candidates that have had refractive surgery after a minimum period of 2 years before application. As each of the 50 brigades in the UK has different requirements, it is best if the applicant contacts them individually to find out the eyesight eligibility criteria.

References

1. Edwards, K. Patient options in vision correction. Optometry Today, 2002.
2. Trends in laser refractive surgery in the UK. Optician 2003;226:12–16.
3. The Royal College of Ophthalmologists. General framework for shared schemes. London: The Royal College of Ophthalmologists,1996.

4. The Association of Optometrists. Primary Care Resource Pack – Establishing co-management schemes. A guide for LOCs and AOCs. London, The Association of Optometrists.
5. The College of Optometrists. Advice for Fellows and Members – Photorefractive Keratectomy. London: The College of Optometrists, 1995.
6. The General Optical Council. Statement on Photorefractive Keratectomy. London: The General Optical Council, 1995.
7. The Royal College of Ophthalmologists. Standards for Laser Refractive Surgery. London: The College of Optometrists, 2003.
8. The General Optical Council. The Rules Relating to Injury or Disease of the Eye. London: The General Optical Council, 1999.
9. The College of Optometrists Member's Handbook. Use of punctal plugs and intra-canalicular occlusion. London: The College of Optometrists.
10. The Prescription Only Medicines (Human use) Order (1997) Schedule 5.
11. The Royal Pharmaceutical Society. Medicines, Ethics and Practice: A Guide for Pharmacists. London: The Royal Pharmaceutical Society.
12. The College of Optometrists Guide. Conducting an emergency examination. London: The College of Optometrists.
13. The British National Formulary. Prescription Writing P.4.
14. The Association of Optometrists Handbook. Advice for members working in refractive surgery.
15. Department of Health. Independent Heathcare National Minimum Care Standards Regulations.
16. The Association of Optometrists Handbook. Occupational Vision Standards.
17. Home Office. Police Officer Eligibility – Eyesight standards.
18. Home Office. Fire Service Circular 9/1996. Visual Standards on the fireground.

Chapter 2

Referral to a laser eye clinic

OVERVIEW

This chapter covers the information that would be useful to an optometrist who wishes to answer a patient's questions about LASIK. It lists the referral criteria and also briefly covers the main contra-indications to surgery. Where the optometrist is referring the patient to a clinic for an initial consultation, details of the patient data that should be forwarded is covered.

CONTENTS

INTRODUCTION

Access to laser eye surgery is widely available and increasing competition between clinics has also made this an affordable option for many more patients. The patient may well contact a clinic directly, but it is likely that they will seek an opinion from a professional that they trust before doing so.

ROUTES OF REFERRAL

Many patients are often emboldened to attend for an initial consultation after a friend or relative has had treatment. Often the patient will attend the same clinic as their friend and will ask to see the same surgeon. Therefore, this route of referral is nurtured by the continuing high standards of care and good surgical results provided by the clinic and the surgeon.

However, some patients will not have the courage to present themselves at a clinic without seeking the advice of their optometrist or general medical practitioner (GP). GPs may not know very much about refractive surgery and are likely to tell the patient to seek the advice of their optometrist. Therefore, it falls on the optometrist to provide the necessary information.

At the end of a normal eye examination, the optometrist usually discusses the appropriate vision correction options for that patient. If the patient is interested in refractive surgery, it is important that the optometrist is able to give accurate and unbiased information. Anecdotal evidence suggests that where the optometrist has been dismissive of this option, the determined patient has sought an alternative source of information. Refractive surgery is now widely available and patients are more likely to stay loyal to a practice if they receive comprehensive advice on all options of vision correction. Below are some patient anecdotes of how they have responded to advice given by their optometrist.

- When asked, an optometrist informed the patient that refractive surgery may be a possibility and that the patient should attend for a consultation with a local laser eye clinic. The patient was found to be suitable and had treatment. The patient still needed varifocals after treatment for VDU and close work and wished to be referred back to this optometrist.

- Another patient refused to have their discharge letter of information sent to their optometrist as the practice had been quite obviously disapproving when he gone in to cancel his contact lens plan. He decided to go elsewhere for his reading spectacles and annual eye examination.

- One patient reported that they had not considered refractive surgery until their local optometrist practice sent out a letter to its patients warning them off refractive surgery.

BASIC CRITERIA FOR SELF REFERRAL

Not all patients are suitable candidates for laser eye surgery. Although each clinic will have individual suitability protocols, the following questions will help the patients to understand if this is an option worth pursuing.

- Is my prescription greater than 1.00 D, and between +5.00 and −9.00 D?
- Has my prescription been stable (*i.e.* changed by less than 0.5 D) over the last 12 months?
- Am I above 21 years of age but less than 65 years.
- Do I have realistic expectations for this type of surgery?
- Am I prepared to sign a consent form for surgery?

If the patients can answer 'yes' to all of the above questions then laser eye surgery may be a suitable option for them.

DETAILED CRITERIA FOR OPTOMETRIST REFERRAL

Patients are usually advised to have an eye examination before booking for an initial consultation with a clinic. If the patient wishes to pursue the refractive surgery option, it will be helpful if the optometrist ensures they are suitable for the initial consultation as some patients may have very obvious reasons for unsuitability. The following findings during an eye examination are indicative of unsuitability for elective refractive surgery.

History and symptoms

Any reported symptoms need to be investigated and resolved prior to refractive surgery. For example, if the patient has flashing lights and floaters, this will need to be investigated and then discharged by an ophthalmologist before refractive surgery can proceed.

Absolute general health contra–indications

Patients in the following categories will not be considered for LASIK.

- **Auto-immune disease** *e.g.* rheumatoid arthritis, systemic lupus erythematosus, thyroid disease – there may be an increased risk of inflammatory complications.[1]

- **Immune suppression** – conditions such as HIV or if the patient is taking immune suppression drugs means that there is an increased risk of infection.

- **Pregnancy** – during pregnancy and lactation the refraction may vary and there is an altered wound healing response. The patient must wait 6 months after giving birth or cessation of breast feeding. This time restriction may vary between clinics.

- **Systemic steroids** – patients that have a condition requiring significant steroid use may also be at a higher risk of developing infections.

- **Amiadarone** – the interaction of the laser with the corneal deposits found with the use of this drug is unknown.

- **5-Hydroxy-tryptamine** *e.g.* sumatriptan – there is an increased risk of vascular occlusion when the intraocular pressure is raised during treatment. The patient can be reconsidered if they are able to change to an alternative drug with the GP's consent for at least 1 month before treatment.

- **Roaccutaine** – this drug causes a significantly decreased tear production. As above, the patient can be considered if the drug is stopped or substituted with the GP's consent for 6 months before treatment.

Relative general health contra-indications

Patients with these relative contra-indications may not be suitable for treatment, but can still attend for the initial consultation. The clinic may require extra information from the patient's GP.

- **Tricyclics or lithium-based medication** – the need for such medication indicates that the patient may have obsessive, compulsive or perfectionist personality traits or is suffering from a significant level of depression. These patients can have expectations of surgery that are too high and are unlikely to be satisfied following surgery. However, care must be taken not to discriminate against such patients and the GP will always be consulted before treatment takes place.

- **Diabetes** – diabetics can have an increased risk of epithelial complications after treatment[2] and so the clinic may require more information about the patient's condition before deciding upon suitability for treatment. Eyes which have signs of diabetic retinopathy are contra-indicated.

- **Active atopy** – any active or uncontrolled atopic disease would be contra-indicated until it is well controlled as it is a risk factor for postoperative inflammation.[3]

- **Epilepsy** – the patient must be able to remain relatively still during the LASIK procedure. Therefore, only patients that have not had an epileptic episode for 12 months or more may be considered for treatment.

- **History of frequent fainting** – these patients may have a low threshold for vasovagal attack. Patients that have a low oculocardiac reflex would also be unsuitable.

- **Hepatitis B and C** – patients with these conditions will not be considered for surgery in many clinics due to the potential risk to surgical staff.

Absolute ocular health contra-indications

- **Diabetic retinopathy** – this is an absolute contra-indication as it can accelerate the progression of diabetic retinopathy. It has also been reported that pronounced aggravation of proliferative retinopathy has occurred after LASIK.[4]

- **Glaucoma** – in eyes which suffer from glaucoma, the optic disc is already compromised. During LASIK treatment, the intraocular pressure (IOP) is raised to above 90 mmHg which may cause further damage to the optic disc. The topical steroids used postoperatively may also affect IOP management in these patients.[5,6]

- **Corneal thinning dystrophies** *e.g.* keratoconus – in dystrophies where the cornea is abnormally thin, LASIK would reduce the corneal thickness even more and may cause keratectasia. Signs of subclinical keratoconus such as inferior steepening of the cornea, even where corneal thickness is adequate are a contra-indication to LASIK.[7,8]

- **History of ocular inflammatory disease** – eyes that have recurrent inflammatory conditions will be more susceptible to inflammatory attack after surgery[1] which may be difficult to control.

- **Herpatic ocular disease** – there is evidence that these inflammatory conditions can be reactivated by laser eye surgery.[9–11]

- **Sjögren's syndrome** – these patients will have acute dry eye and their symptoms will be exacerbated by treatment.

- **Fuch's endothelial dystrophy** – endothelial decompensation and poor flap adhesion has been associated with this condition.[12,13]

- **Unstable refractive error** – the prescription must be fairly stable before treatment is considered. A change of more the 0.50 D equivalent in 12 months or less is deemed unstable. In come cases, the clinic may request copies of the spectacle prescriptions from the previous 3 years to ensure stability.

- **Visually significant cataract** – in cases where there is a significant lens opacity, it is in the patient's best interest that this be treated first. Further refractive surgery afterwards may or may not be necessary.

Relative ocular health contra-indications

- **Dry eye** – in some patients their condition may be temporarily worse after treatment. In patients where the dry eye is mild, it is unlikely to interfere with their suitability. The clinic will decide on a case-by-case basis those whom are suitable for treatment.

- **Blepharitis** – all signs of blepharitis must be absent prior to treatment as it may induce postoperative inflammation.[14] The surgeon may expect the patient to adopt lid hygiene measures and in some cases use medication for several weeks prior treatment.

- **Nystagmus** – not all lasers have a tracker that can keep up with the involuntary eye movements associated with nystagmus. It is best to contact the clinic direct prior to referring the patient.

Contra-indicated eye examination findings

- **Unaided vision** – patients with very good unaided vision and who only need spectacles to correct presbyopia are not suitable for treatment in most cases. In some instances, monovision may be an acceptable option after careful discussion with the surgeon. Many surgeons will not consider making an emmetropic eye myopic to create monovision.

- **Binocular vision status** – if the patient has prism controlled diplopia or where decompensated heterophoria is corrected by the use of prism in spectacles, refractive surgery may not be suitable as it does not correct this element of the spectacle prescription. Therefore, prismatic correction may still be needed after treatment. For some patients, this is not an acceptable outcome.

- **Refraction** – most clinics will treat a myopic range of -0.75 to -9.00 D. Anything less is probably not visually significant enough to justify treatment. The hypermetropic range is much narrower and most clinics will treat between $+1.00$ and $+4.00$ D. LASIK can also successfully treat astigmatism and clinics will often treat up to -4.00 DC. Prescriptions outside of this range are usually contraindicated for LASIK as the results are less predictable. The above prescription ranges refer to the highest powered meridian; for example, a prescription of $-8.00/-3.00 \times 180$ would not be suitable as the most myopic meridian is -11.00 D.

- **Best corrected visual acuity (BCVA)** – in cases of significant amblyopia where the BCVA of the amblyopic eye is less than 6/12, treatment of the other eye will be contra-indicated. Where no amblyopia exists, but the binocular BCVA is 6/9 or less, treatment may still be contra-indicated as there is a small risk of loss of one or two lines of BCVA after treatment.

- **Near vision** – presbyopic patients must understand that reading spectacles will still be necessary after LASIK to correct their distance vision unless they opt for monovision. For myopes, this means deliberate undercorrection of the less dominant eye. For hypermetropes it would mean overcorrection, which will probably worsen the unaided distance vision in the eye that has been corrected for near vision tasks. If the patient refuses to accept these options, then they are not suitable for LASIK.

INFORMATION TO SEND TO THE CLINIC

The following information may be useful for the clinic when assessing the patient's suitability for treatment.

Referral to Laser Eye Clinic

Practice/Clinic Name:
Address:
Telephone Nos:

Date:

Re: Px Name: DOB:
      Px Address:

The above patient is considering laser eye surgery. The following information may be of use in deciding suitability for treatment.

Date of most recent eye examination:

Refraction			VA	Near Add	NVA
R:	/	/	6/	+	N
L:	/	/	6/	+	N

Previous prescriptions:
Date:

Refraction			VA	Near Add	NVA
R:	/	/	6/	+	N
L:	/	/	6/	+	N

Date:

Refraction			VA	Near Add	NVA
R:	/	/	6/	+	N
L:	/	/	6/	+	N

Current contact lens prescription:
Date:

Lens Type	BOZR	TD	Lens power
R:	/	/	/
L:	/	/	/

Baseline Keratometry readings:

R:	mm@	mm@
L:	mm@	mm@

Relevant medical/ocular history:

Other information:

Yours faithfully,

Figure 2.1   A typical referral report to a laser eye clinic

- Copies of the prescription with visual acuity measurements from the last 3 eye examinations.
- Current contact lens prescription where applicable.
- Baseline keratometry readings taken at initial contact lens fitting if available.
- Details of any medical or ocular history that may affect suitability for treatment.

An example of a typical referral report to a clinic can be seen in Figure 2.1. A blank copy can also be printed off from <www.optometryonline.net>. The patient must consent to the sharing of their clinical information that is detailed in the referral report.

PREPARING THE PATIENT FOR CONSULTATION

Some clinics provide written information for the patient to read prior to attending for consultation. This information is also widely available in optometry practices where the practitioner is part of a co-management scheme. Some optometrists prefer not to refer to any particular clinic or may not have this information available to hand out.

The following instructions are important for any patient intending to attend for a consultation. A printable version is available at <www.optometryonline.net> which can be given to the patient.

- Soft contact lens wearers need to leave their lenses out for a minimum of 1 week. Rigid lens wearers must leave lenses out for at least 2 weeks. If they are aware of some spectacle blur after removing their lenses it would be advisable to leave the lenses out for 4 weeks prior to consultation.

- Eyedrops may be administered to dilate the pupils or to carry out a cycloplegic refraction. Therefore, the patient should come accompanied to the clinic if possible as it will not be safe for them to drive home afterwards. They may also wish to bring sunglasses to avoid discomfort glare after dilation.

- Patients who are on medication are advised to bring a list of their medications with them.

- Patients should be advised to allow up to 2 hours for the consultation.

PROCEDURES THAT THE PATIENT CAN EXPECT

Patients may be apprehensive about attending a laser eye clinic and so informing them of what to expect may help. There can be differences between the way various clinics carry out consultations with some being ophthalmologist led and others being with an optometrist only. However, most clinics will perform a similar battery of tests and data collection procedures to assess the patient suitability for treatment.

- **Vision assessment** – the level of vision achieved with and without spectacle correction.
- **Refraction** – manifest and cycloplegic refraction where necessary.
- **Focimetry of spectacles** – together with the refraction results, it can be used to check prescription stability over a period of time.
- **Binocular vision assessment** – the evaluation of any potential issues that may arise from existing anomalies after treatment.
- **Ocular dominance testing** – this is carried out on all patients but is particularly relevant with presbyopic patients who are considering monovision.
- **Tonometry** – the IOP is measured as part of the examination to check for suitability for treatment. The information is also useful baseline data, as the measured IOP can change after treatment.
- **Tear film assessment** – the patient's tear quality and quantity will be evaluated to identify and to advise patients that are more susceptible to dry eye after treatment.
- **Anterior eye examination and dilated fundoscopy** – an assessment of the ocular structures to ensure that there are no contra-indicated features.
- **Pupillometry** – the pupil size in scotopic conditions is measured and is taken into consideration when deciding upon the treatment zone size.
- **Pachymetry** – the corneal thickness is measured and a calculation is carried out to find out whether the patient's prescription can be corrected on their eyes with LASIK.
- **Topography** – this will provide a visual map showing the contours of the anterior surface of the cornea. Some clinics may also have equipment to map out the posterior surface. It is primarily used to screen for corneal anomalies.
- **Wavefront aberrometry** – this is used in some clinics to measure the optical aberrations of the eye. It is used to identify those patients that may have an increased susceptibility to visually significant higher order aberrations after LASIK.

FURTHER PATIENT INFORMATION

Some patients may feel bewildered by the choice of clinics and procedures available to them. If they decide to attend for an initial consultation, they may wish to ask lots of questions about the procedure and the potential complications with LASIK. It is important that they choose a clinic or a surgeon that they trust.

LASIK requires the use of a microkeratome and The Royal College of Ophthalmologists' guidelines for best clinical practice state that: 'only surgeons registered with the General Medical Council as ophthalmic specialists who have also undertaken a period of training in automated lamellar surgery, should perform this procedure'.[15]

In a guide for patients issued by The Royal College of Ophthalmologists on laser photorefractive surgery, it is recommended that refractive surgeons are fully trained ophthalmologists that have undergone specialist training in refractive surgery. It also recommends that patients check that the clinic they choose adheres to the *Guidelines for Laser Refractive Surgery* of The Royal College of Ophthalmologists.[16]

References

1. Lahners WJ, Hardten DR, Lindstrom RL. Peripheral keratitis following laser *in situ* keratomileusis. J Refract Surg 2003;19:671–675.
2. Fraunfelder FW, Rich LF. Laser-assisted *in situ* keratomileusis complications in diabetes mellitus. Cornea 2002;21:246–248.
3. Boorstein SM, Henk HJ, Elner VM. Atopy: a patient-specific risk factor for diffuse lamellar keratitis. Ophthalmology 2003;110:131–137.
4. Ghanbari H, Ahmadieh H. Aggravation of proliferative diabetic retinopathy after laser *in situ* keratomileusis. J Cataract Refract Surg 2003;29:2232–2233.
5. Davidson RS, Brandt JD, Mannis MJ. Intraocular pressure-induced interlamellar keratitis after LASIK surgery. J Glaucoma 2003;12:23–26.
6. Shaikh NM, Shaikh S, Singh K *et al.* Progression to end-stage glaucoma after laser *in situ* keratomileusis. J Cataract Refract Surg 2002;28:356–359.
7. Chiang RK, Park AJ, Rapuano CJ *et al.* Bilateral keratoconus after LASIK in a keratoconus patient. Eye Contact Lens 2003;29:90–92.
8. Randleman JB, Russell B, Ward MA *et al.* Risk factors and prognosis for corneal ectasia after LASIK. Ophthalmology 2003;110:267–275.
9. Perry HD, Doshi SJ, Donnenfeld ED *et al.* Herpes simplex reactivation following laser *in situ* keratomileusis and subsequent corneal perforation. CLAO J 2002;28:69–71.
10. Jarade EF, Tabbara KF. Presumed reactivation of herpes zoster ophthalmicus following laser *in situ* keratomileusis. J Refract Surg 2002;18:79–80.
11. Dhaliwal DK, Romanowski EG, Yates KA *et al.* Experimental laser-assisted *in situ* keratomileusis induces the reactivation of latent herpes simplex virus. Am J Ophthalmol 2001;131:506–507.
12. Dastjerdi MH, Sugar A. Corneal decompensation after laser *in situ* keratomileusis in Fuch's endothelial dystrophy. Cornea 2003;22:379–381.
13. Vroman DT, Solomon KD, Holzer MP *et al.* Endothelial decompensation after laser *in situ* keratomileusis. J Cataract Refract Surg 2002;28:2045–2049.
14. Ambrosio Jr R, Periman LM, Netto MV *et al.* Bilateral marginal sterile infiltrates and diffuse lamellar keratitis after laser *in situ* keratomileusis. J Refract Surg 2003;19:154–158.
15. The Royal College of Ophthalmologists. Excimer laser photo-ablative surgery: best clinical practice guidelines. London: The Royal College of Ophthalmologists, 1998.
16. The Royal College of Ophthalmologists. A patient's guide to excimer laser photorefractive surgery. London: The Royal College of Ophthalmologists, 2003.

Chapter **3**

Pre-operative assessment – data collection

OVERVIEW

This chapter considers data collection aspects of the pre-operative assessment. Information is provided to aid the interpretation of data collected, and this is then related to relevant aspects of the treatment procedure.

CONTENTS

INTRODUCTION

The purpose of the pre-operative assessment is:

- To determine by physical measurement whether it is possible to correct a patient's individual refractive error on their eyes.
- To determine by examination whether the ocular health is adequate for this procedure.
- To identify if there is any increased risk of complications specific to that patient.
- To allow the patient to have any questions or concerns addressed.

KERATOMETRY

Keratometry (K) readings provide important information about the shape of the cornea. Optometrists and contact lens opticians are familiar with K readings in millimetre units whereas ophthalmologists record K readings in dioptres. Where the K readings are below 41 D or greater than 46 D, there is a greater risk of microkeratome complications and the patient needs to be warned accordingly.

If the cornea is too steep or too flat after treatment severe aberrations may be induced. Where the postoperative cornea is less than 35 D or greater than 50 D, aberrations can disable vision significantly. This would be particularly problematic at night when the pupil dilates. These patients should be carefully evaluated by the surgeon before treatment. In some cases, the patient may be deemed unsuitable.

The keratometry mires (Figure 3.1) are also useful as they indicate if there is any irregular astigmatism on the visual axis. The K readings will also indicate the degree of corneal astigmatism which can be compared to the refractive error. Where significant lenticular astigmatism is found, it is necessary to inform the patient that if corneal surgery compensates this error, further astigmatic correction may be required should they require cataract surgery in the future. It is also important to record the K readings as baseline data. This information would be useful should the patient need an intraocular lens implant in the future and should be included in their discharge information to their doctor or optometrist.

TOPOGRAPHY

This analysis is essential in assessing the suitability of the patient's eye for treatment. Keratometry gives a limited amount of information as it only measures 4 points within the central 3 or 4 mm of the cornea, whereas topographers can evaluate up to 11 000 points across the entire corneal surface. Together with computer software and imagery, it provides significantly more detailed information about the entire corneal surface, not just the central area.

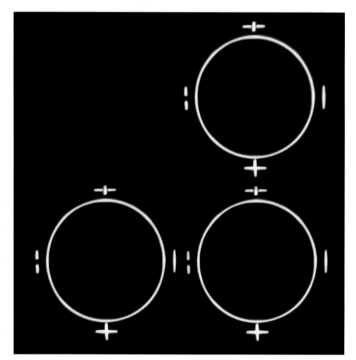

Figure 3.1   Keratometry mires as viewed with a Bausch & Lomb keratometer

Topography is used in the pre-operative assessment to screen for anterior corneal surface anomalies that may interfere with or contra-indicate treatment. It is also useful in monitoring the progression of a patient who has had corneal surgery. Any changes to the corneal shape after treatment and as it recovers from surgery will be evident from topographical analysis.

Types of topographic displays

Topography instruments have become increasingly sophisticated and most are able to present several displays.

Axial map   This is a simple display which assumes that the eye is spherical. It displays the corneal surface as a topographical map where the colours of the map indicate the dioptric power of the cornea. The flatter areas are shown in 'cool' colours such as blue and green and the steeper areas are shown in 'hot' colours such as red and orange. Although easy to interpret, this map tends to 'smooth out' some of the smaller areas of curvature variation. Figure 3.2a shows an axial map of an astigmatic eye. There is a vertical bow-tie appearance which is typical of rule astigmatism.

Tangential map   This map uses colours in the same way as the axial map to display dioptric power but uses a different algorithm to calculate the corneal

(a)

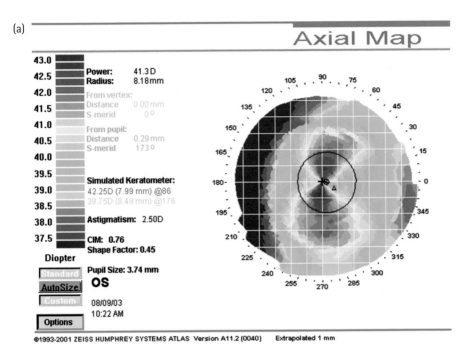

Axial Map

Diopter	
43.0	
42.5	
42.0	
41.5	
41.0	
40.5	
40.0	
39.5	
39.0	
38.5	
38.0	
37.5	

Power: 41.3 D
Radius: 8.18 mm
From vertex:
Distance 0.00 mm
S-merid 0°
From pupil:
Distance 0.29 mm
S-merid 173°

Simulated Keratometer:
42.25D (7.99 mm) @86
39.75D (8.49 mm) @176

Astigmatism: 2.50D

CIM: 0.76
Shape Factor: 0.45

Pupil Size: 3.74 mm
Standard
AutoSize
Custom
Options

OS

08/09/03
10:22 AM

©1993-2001 ZEISS HUMPHREY SYSTEMS ATLAS Version A11.2 (0040) Extrapolated 1 mm

(b)

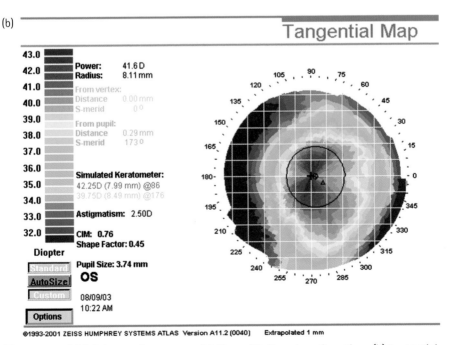

Tangential Map

Diopter	
43.0	
42.0	
41.0	
40.0	
39.0	
38.0	
37.0	
36.0	
35.0	
34.0	
33.0	
32.0	

Power: 41.6 D
Radius: 8.11 mm
From vertex:
Distance 0.00 mm
S-merid 0°
From pupil:
Distance 0.29 mm
S-merid 173°

Simulated Keratometer:
42.25D (7.99 mm) @86
39.75D (8.49 mm) @176

Astigmatism: 2.50D

CIM: 0.76
Shape Factor: 0.45

Pupil Size: 3.74 mm
Standard
AutoSize
Custom
Options

OS

08/09/03
10:22 AM

©1993-2001 ZEISS HUMPHREY SYSTEMS ATLAS Version A11.2 (0040) Extrapolated 1 mm

Figure 3.2 (a) Axial map of a cornea exhibiting with the rule astigmatism; (b) tangential display of the same eye (*continued on next page*)

(c)

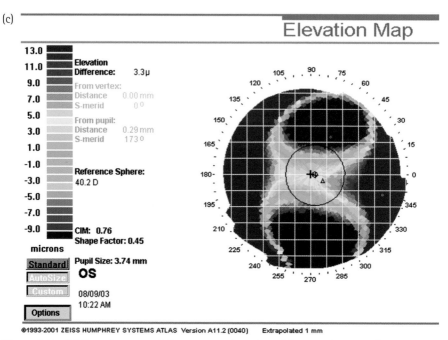

Figure 3.2 (c) Elevation map of the same eye (*continued from previous page*)

curvature and is able to map the peripheral curves of the cornea more accurately. It does not assume that the eye is spherical but bases its calculations on the local curvature at a given meridian. This display represents the 'true' corneal profile and is able to show sharp power transitions more easily than the axial map. It is very useful for showing the changes that occur as the cornea heals postoperatively. Figure 3.2b shows the same eye using a tangential display which shows the true curvature of the eye.

Elevation map   Figure 3.2c shows the measured height from which the corneal curvature varies from a computer-selected reference surface. Warm colours indicate points above the reference line and cool colours represent points below. This display is useful in evaluating corneal irregularities and post-surgical abnormalities.

Photokeratoscopic view   This is an actual image of the eye that is captured by the video camera. The tear film acts like a convex mirror and reflects the illuminated placido rings (Figure 3.3a). The spacing between the concentric rings can indicate the steepness of the cornea if there are gross changes. Any irregularity of the mires can indicate corneal distortion or where the tear film has evaporated. This information can be useful in ruling out artefacts on maps caused by factors such as dry eye. In Figure 3.3b, the axial map of the cornea looks slightly unusual nasally. The reason for this can be seen in the photokeratoscopic image (Figure 3.3c) which shows corneal distortion that is caused by a pterygium encroaching the cornea.

Topography scales

When interpreting maps, it is imperative that the practitioner refers to the scale of the map before drawing conclusions. There are generally two types of scale that are commonly used.

(a)

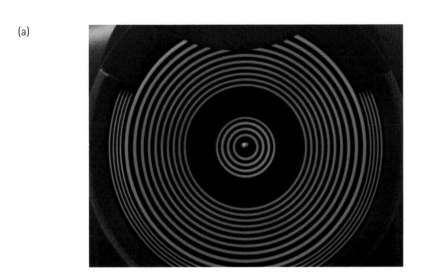

(b)

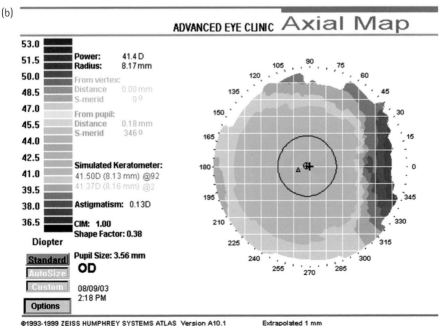

Figure 3.3 (a) Photograph of the placido rings that are projected onto the cornea; (b) nasal corneal irregularity with apparent flattening (*continued on next page*)

(c)

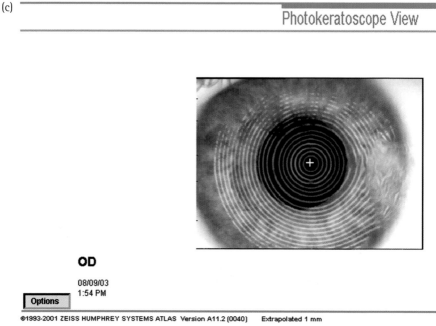

Photokeratoscope View

OD

08/09/03
1:54 PM

Options

©1993-2001 ZEISS HUMPHREY SYSTEMS ATLAS Version A11.2 (0040)   Extrapolated 1 mm

Figure 3.3 (c) Photograph of the projected placido rings show that the irregularity is due to the presence of a pterygium (*continued from previous page*)

Absolute scale This is a fixed numerical scale where each colour represents a specified dioptric power. The range of the scale is the same for each map. This scale is useful in the general screening for anomalies as only features of clinical significance will be visible. Although specific corneal anomalies appear more subtle with an absolute scale, the practitioner will be able to interpret the maps more easily with experience. Figure 3.4a shows the same eye as in Figure 3.2 but uses an absolute scale rather than a normalised one. The plots look quite different, but the actual data are the same. The benefit of a fixed scale is the easy comparison of different maps. Comparison between maps from the eyes of a patient is straightforward using an absolute scale and it can be seen in Figure 3.4b that the eyes are fairly symmetrical and both have oblique astigmatism.

Normalised scale This is a floating scale where the computer selects the numerical range from the highest and lowest data points. Therefore, the colours of the map will show a very detailed display of the cornea. Every small curvature change will be detectable; as a result, it may introduce a significant amount of 'noise' which could mislead the practitioner. As the scale is relative to that particular cornea, it can be difficult to compare multiple maps or to track the progress of corneal changes. However, if a condition is detected with the absolute scale, the detail given on a normalised can be useful for further analysis of that condition. Figure 3.5a shows a suspect keratoconus that is detectable on an absolute scale, but more detailed information is seen with the normalised scale (Figure 3.5b).

(a)

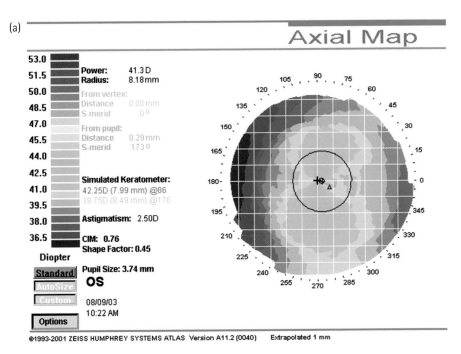

(b)

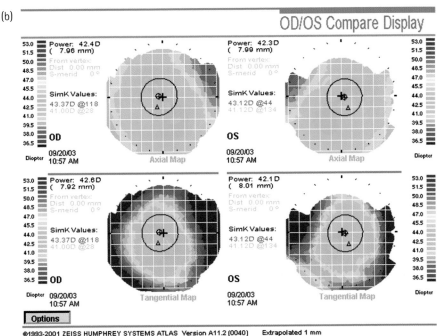

Figure 3.4   (a) Map of an astigmatic cornea presented with an absolute scale; (b) comparison of multiple maps is facilitated by using an absolute scale (*continued on next page*)

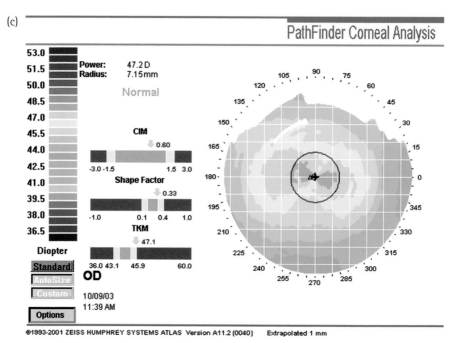

Figure 3.4   (c) Against the rule astigmatism (*continued from previous page*)

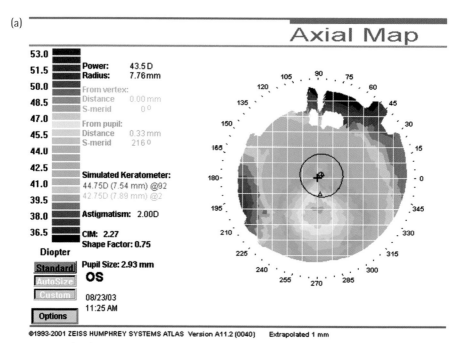

Figure 3.5   (a, b) A keratoconus suspect – the use of different scales can be used to screen or investigate conditions (*continued on next page*)

(b)

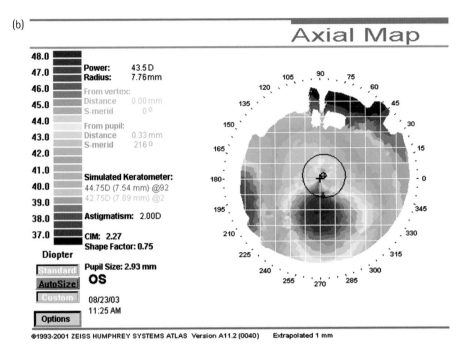

Axial Map

Power: 43.5 D
Radius: 7.76 mm

From vertex:
Distance   0.00 mm
S-merid   0°

From pupil:
Distance   0.33 mm
S-merid   216°

Simulated Keratometer:
44.75D (7.54 mm) @92
42.75D (7.89 mm) @2

Astigmatism: 2.00D

CIM: 2.27
Shape Factor: 0.75

Diopter

Standard
AutoSize
Custom
Options

Pupil Size: 2.93 mm

OS

08/23/03
11:25 AM

©1993-2001 ZEISS HUMPHREY SYSTEMS ATLAS Version A11.2 (0040)   Extrapolated 1 mm

(c)

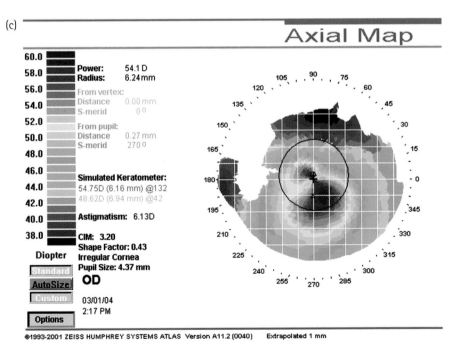

Axial Map

Power: 54.1 D
Radius: 6.24 mm

From vertex:
Distance   0.00 mm
S-merid   0°

From pupil:
Distance   0.27 mm
S-merid   270°

Simulated Keratometer:
54.75D (6.16 mm) @132
48.62D (6.94 mm) @42

Astigmatism: 6.13D

CIM: 3.20
Shape Factor: 0.43
Irregular Cornea

Diopter

Standard
AutoSize
Custom
Options

Pupil Size: 4.37 mm

OD

03/01/04
2:17 PM

©1993-2001 ZEISS HUMPHREY SYSTEMS ATLAS Version A11.2 (0040)   Extrapolated 1 mm

Figure 3.5   (c) Moderate keratoconus where the corneal curvature is greater than 55 D at the apex of the cone (*continued from previous page*)

Map interpretation

The colours of a topography map can be misleading and to avoid misinterpretation of the data it is important to have a systematic approach.

1. The first and most obvious step is to confirm that the patient details correspond with the patient that is being examined.
2. Check the type of map being shown.
3. Check the type of scale being used and the step interval used between colours.
4. Check the dioptric powers on the map and see if they fall with the normal range. Readings of 47 D or greater are suspicious and could indicate keratoconus.
5. Look of areas of unusual flattening or steepening as well as any asymmetry.
6. Look for features that would identify specific conditions.

Chart 3.1 shows a decision-making flow chart to aid interpretation of topography maps and to reach a clinical decision.

The following section describes the features that are commonly seen in the pre-operative screening of patients for corneal abnormalities. There are other corneal disorders that are not mentioned here and further information is available from other texts on topography.

The normal cornea   The normal cornea is prolate in shape, meaning it is steeper in the centre and flatter towards the periphery. It should be reasonably uniform in appearance with a dioptic power of 42–46 D at the centre. As the cornea flattens towards the periphery, the dioptric power declines and the nasal cornea shows a greater degree of change than the temporal cornea. Normal corneas may also have a small astigmatic component and there is usually a degree of mirror image symmetry between the two eyes.

The astigmatic eye   In most cases the astigmatism is regular, with the steepest and the flattest meridians at 90° to each other. Astigmatism typically looks like a 'bow tie' or a figure of eight on a topography map. Where the steeper meridian is vertical, it is called 'With the Rule' (see Figures 3.2a and 3.4a) as it the most common form of astigmatism. 'Against the Rule' astigmatism has the steeper meridian in the horizontal position (Figure 3.4c). An example of oblique astigmatism can be seen in Figure 3.4b, where the axis of the cylinder is near to 45° or 135°.

Keratoconus   This is characterised by inferior localised steepening of the cornea. The example shown in Figure 3.5a,b is a mild form of keratoconus where the maximum dioptric power of the cornea is less than 55 D. The apex of the cone is usually found slightly to the left or right of the 6-o'clock position as in Figure 3.5c, which is also a more significant degree of keratoconus. The map is displayed using a normalised scale as the standard scale is not large enough to cover the dioptric range of the cornea. Keratoconus can also be classified according location and shape of the cone.

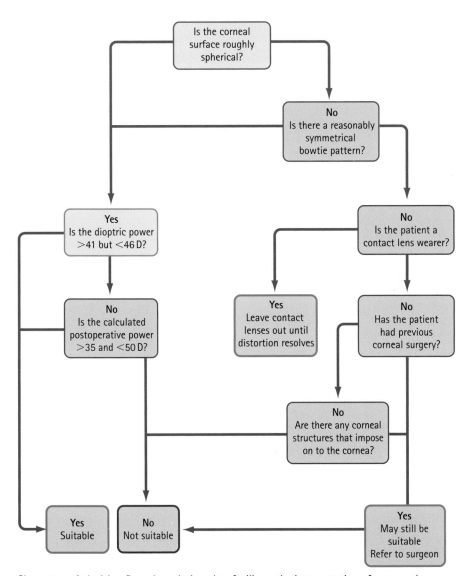

Chart 3.1 A decision flow chart designed to facilitate the interpretation of topography maps

Pterygium This is an anomaly in which a triangular formation of tissue extends from the nasal conjunctiva towards the limbus. In advanced cases, it also encroaches the cornea and extends towards the central cornea. This can cause some flattening out of the cornea as shown in Figure 3.3b.

Contact lens induced distortion Contact lens wearers are asked to keep their contact lenses out for between 1 and 4 weeks depending upon their type of lens and their wearing habits. This is due to the possibility of some lenses causing corneal distortion. In some cases, this rest period is not long enough and distortion can still be seen. In other cases the patient simply has not followed instructions. Where corneal distortion is found in a contact lens wearer, it is necessary to repeat topography at suitable intervals until the distortion disappears.

In some cases, the warpage can mimic keratoconus with the exception that the overall corneal power is usually below 46 D. The warpage also tends to be more elongated than circular.[1] Figure 3.6a shows an example of peripheral steepening, where there is a localised area of inferior temporal cornea steepening outside of the lens margin. Other forms of contact lens induced warpage include central flattening and furrow depression. Apparent corneal distortion can also occur when localised patches of the tear film break up. Topography needs to be repeated after instilling a rewetting drop.

Other presentations

Refractive map   This shows the true refractive state of the cornea which can be useful in determining the outcome of a corneal refractive procedure. It can also be used to evaluate the visual performance in eyes that have had a procedure already. The calculation used to produce this map takes spherical aberration and corneal asphericity into account and is able to show the true dioptric power of the eye.

Corneal analysis   Many topographers now have sophisticated software that is designed to differentiate between normal and abnormal corneas. The images in Figure 3.6 taken with The Humphrey® Atlas™ Corneal Topographer have been analysed using the Mastervue™ software. The program has three corneal indices which give an overview of the corneal shape:

- **Corneal irregularity measurement** (CIM) – This number represents the irregularity of the corneal surface in comparison to a perfect model toric cornea. The index is able to highlight irregularities such as contact lens warpage and irregular astigmatism.
- **Shape factor** (SF) – This is a measurement which accounts for the asphericity of the cornea, where an index is assigned to represent the shape of that surface.
- **Mean toric keratometry** (MTK) – This is a mean value of apical curvature where a high value would indicate an excessively toric cornea.

The indices are shown on the left, with the normal range indicated on the bar in green. The yellow and red areas represent borderline and abnormal measurements respectively. It can be seen in Figure 3.6a that although the CIM is within normal range, the SF and the MTK are in the abnormal range. However, the software cannot replace clinical judgement as demonstrated in Figure 3.6b. Subclinical keratoconus is indicated but the location and shape of the distortion is more indicative of contact lens induced warpage.

Profile views   Further information can be obtained by looking at a profile of the cornea. Figure 3.7a is profile view of the suspect keratoconus shown in

(a)
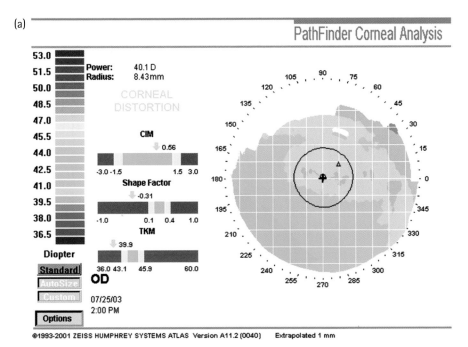

(b)
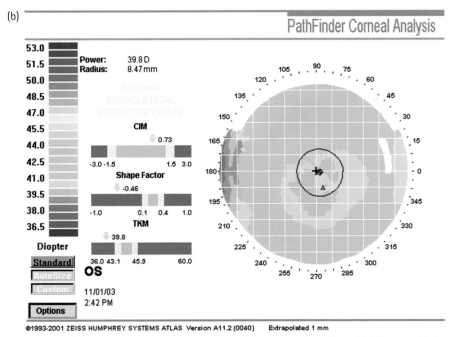

Figure 3.6 (a) Contact lens induced distortion; (b) corneal distortion which is more likely to be due to contact lens wear rather than subclinical keratoconus

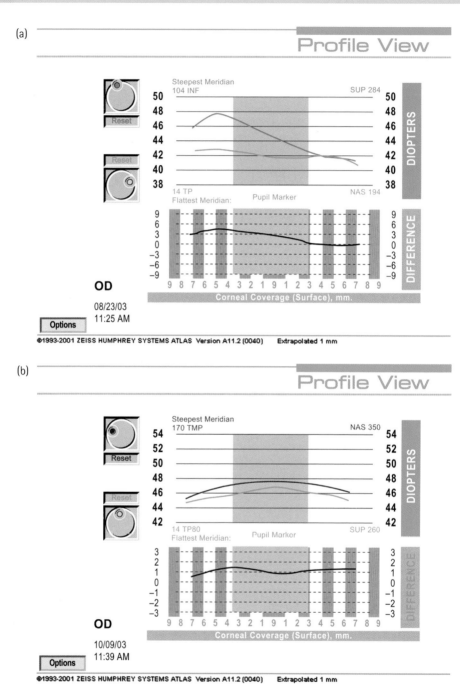

Figure 3.7   Further data analysis programs can give more details about the corneal curvature characteristics: (a) keratoconic profile; (b) normal astigmatic profile

Figure 3.5. At a glance, it informs the examiner the dioptric power and the axes of the principal meridians. It shows that the astigmatism is not symmetrical on the cornea unlike in the eye with ATR astigmatism shown in Figure 3.7b.

TOMOGRAPHY

The Orbscan II tomographer is the only instrument that is currently able to produce an elevation map of the posterior corneal surface. It uses a scanning slit to collect information from both the anterior and posterior surfaces of the cornea. The information is then processed by the instrument to generate elevation maps of the corneal surfaces (see Figure 3.8a). A 'posterior float' of more than 0.05 mm is considered suspicious and contra-indicates LASIK. It is useful in detecting those corneas which may be at higher risk of keratoconus or kerectasia after surgery. The Orbscan II is also able to produce other data such as corneal thickness as indicated in Figure 3.8b. Studies have shown that pachymetry readings taken by this method have good correlation with traditional ultrasound pachymetry on untreated corneas.[2–5]

PUPILLOMETRY

Accurate pupil measurement is an absolute necessity prior to corneal laser surgery as 1 mm can make a huge difference to the amount of tissue that needs to be ablated. For example, using the Munnerlyn formula, a -5.00 D error requires a 60 µm ablation depth using a 6 mm treatment zone, whereas a 7 mm zone requires an ablation depth of 81.7 µm.

The evaluation of pupil size should be carried out under mesopic and scotopic light conditions. The data are used to select an appropriate ablation zone diameter. After refractive surgery, visual quality can be significantly influenced by the size of the pupil, so the size of the treatment zone is usually set so that the effective optic zone diameter is greater than the scotopic pupil diameter. This is necessary to minimise the risk of glare, ghosting and haloing after treatment.

The greater the pupil diameter, the greater the ablation zone size and the greater the amount of corneal tissue that is removed. This may render some eyes unsuitable for treatment as a stromal bed thickness of 250 µm must remain after treatment to minimise the risk of ectasia. Where the ablation zone needs to be smaller than the scotopic pupil, it may be possible to create a blend zone where the area between the treated and untreated cornea. This lessens the risk of visual disturbance postoperatively.

Methods of pupil measurement

Topography   Many topographers measure the pupil diameter; but, as the instrument uses some light to take its measurements, it cannot be related to real-life conditions reliably.

(a)
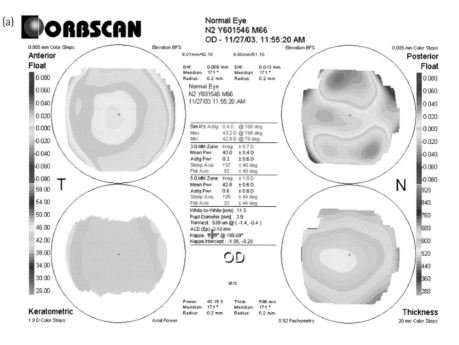

(b)
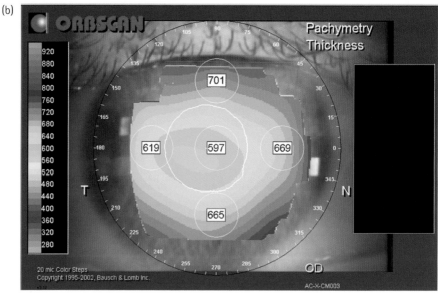

Figure 3.8   (a) Corneal data of a normal eye collected by an Orbscan tomographer; (b) pachymetry map of a cornea (more measurements can be displayed if required). (Reproduced with permission of Bausch & Lomb UK Ltd)

Direct comparison (Morton's pupillometer) A strip with calibrated holes of increasing size can be held up in front of the patient's eye until a match is found.

Projection method (Magnani's pupillometer) An image of the pupil under normal lighting conditions is projected onto a graduated grid.

Light amplification pupillometry (Colvard pupillometer) The room illumination is turned down and the pupil diameter is measured under low-light conditions which simulates the light conditions of night driving. The pupil is viewed through the instrument (see Figure 3.9a) via a phosphorescent screen which intensifies the image. A graduated grid is projected over the image obtained so that a measurement can be taken.

Infrared dynamic pupillometry (Procyon dynamic pupillometer) This is an objective measurement of the pupil diameter under different lighting conditions. The instrument uses a video camera to capture images of both pupils simultaneously, then uses a mathematical 'best fit' analysis to calculate the pupil size. The instrument is able to capture up to 32 frames at a rate of 5 frames per second in mesopic and scotopic conditions, thus increasing the reliability of the final measurement. Figure 3.9b shows frames that were captured under various lighting conditions and it can be seen at a glance that there is also some asymmetry between the eyes. The average from each set of frames is calculated and presented to the instrument operator in a table. An experienced operator is also able to analyse each frame individually and erase any erroneous ones to maximise accuracy.

(a)

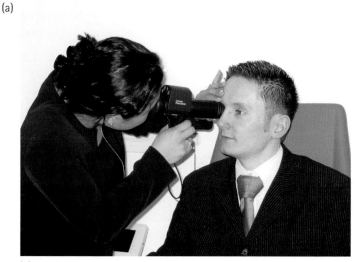

Figure 3.9 (a) Light amplification pupillometry using the Colvard pupillometer
(*continued on next page*)

(b) Mesopic

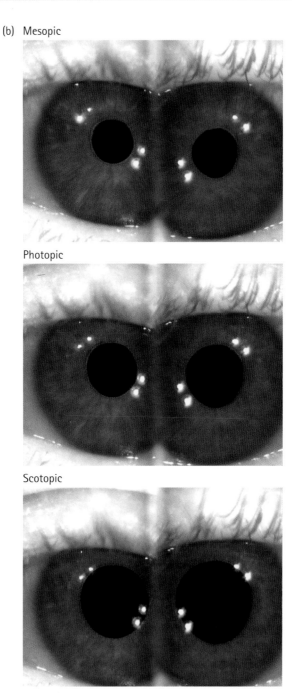

Photopic

Scotopic

Figure 3.9   (b) Captured images of the pupils using the Procyon pupillometer: pupils viewed in mesopic, photopic and scotopic lighting conditions as indicated (*continued from previous page*)

Selecting treatment zone size

This parameter is ultimately decided upon by the treating surgeon; however, it is necessary for the optometrist to select a provisional treatment zone size in order to carry out the suitability calculation. The effective optic zone after treatment is smaller than the actual ablation zone due to the oblate corneal profile created by surgery.[6] This effect increases with the amount of corrected refractive error and with hypermetropic corrections. Ideally, the treatment zone should be greater than the scotopic pupil and be as big as possible to minimise the risks of visual disturbance associated with glare. However, this is constrained by the corneal thickness and the refractive error to be corrected.

In some cases, it may be necessary to select a treatment zone that is smaller than the scotopic pupil to provide the requested correction and maintain the required stromal thickness. In such cases, the patient needs to be warned of the increased possibility of glare in dim illumination. The glare effects can be reduced in such cases by incorporating a blend zone to minimise the effect of the transition between treated and untreated cornea which steepens with increasing corrected refractive error.

WAVEFRONT ABERROMETRY

Wavefront aberrometry is a method of measuring the optical aberrations of the eye. A wave of light from a laser beam is sent through the eye to the retina and is reflected back through the pupil. A sensor detects the reflected wavefront and an aberrometer compares it to an ideal wavefront. The differences detected show the aberrations that are present in the eye's visual system and can be displayed as a three dimensional map (Figure 3.10a). Lower order aberrations such a spherical and astigmatic error are detected as well as higher order aberrations such as coma. The wavefront data can be used to program the laser to reshape the cornea using a customised ablation for each individual eye. Theoretically, this could correct all the aberrations of the eye, not just refractive error.

Wavefront information has been used successfully in astronomy to improve image quality in telescopes, but it has not had the same success with corneal ablation so far. The reason for this is that the cornea is a biomechanical structure that changes in response to treatment. Wavefront sensors do not provide information outside of the pupil, but factors which influence the corneal shape outside the pupil can also affect the cornea inside the pupil. Therefore, the aberrations that are measured in the preoperative cornea can be very different to the postoperative cornea and new aberrations may be induced or existing aberrations exacerbated. As technology improves, the outcomes of wavefront guided ablations are also improving. The risk of higher order aberrations that exists with conventional LASIK can be much lower with appropriate wavefront guided ablation.

Wavefront analysis gives more information about the aberration of the eye than any other system. It can detect those patients who have higher order aberrations that cannot be corrected with surgery or that may be exacerbated by conventional treatment. It is, therefore, an invaluable diagnostic tool. Figure 3.10b

(a)

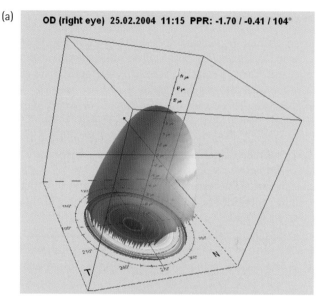

(b)

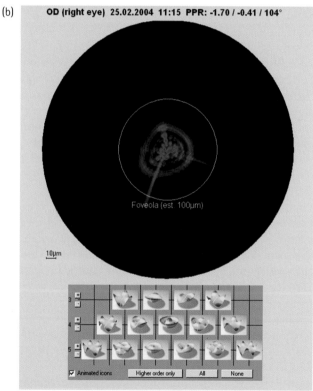

Figure 3.10   (a) Wavefront aberrometry 3-D display; (b) aberration of a point source in an untreated eye (*continued on next page*)

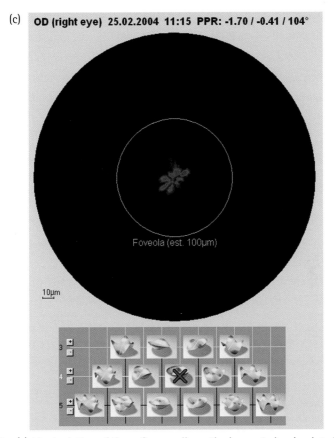

(c)   OD (right eye) 25.02.2004 11:15 PPR: -1.70 / -0.41 / 104°

Figure 3.10   (c) Manipulation of the software allows the image to be simulated with selected aberrations removed (*continued from previous page*)

shows significant aberration in a pre-operative eye. It can be seen in Figure 3.10c that by removing the spherical aberration, the remaining aberrations are much less, but significant higher order aberrations can be seen (greater than 0.30 μm). This patient may, therefore, benefit from customised ablation.

Wavefront-guided ablations could potentially improve the visual outcomes of corneal refractive surgery as well as correct night vision disturbances caused by previous corneal surgery. The advantages of wavefront guided ablation include:

- Potentially increased probability of achieving an acuity 6/6 or better without spectacles.
- Potentially reduced risk of losing best corrected visual acuity and of night vision problems (such as glare and reduced contrast sensitivity).

There are also other factors that need to be considered apart from the actual aberrations. Kezirian, an ophthalmologist working with a refractive surgery software development company, analysed the outcomes of several wavefront platforms. His advice on when to choose wavefront guided ablation over conventional ablation can be summarised into 4 key observations.[7] If the following observations were found, customised ablation would not be indicated.

- Where the aberrometer refraction differs from the manifest refraction more than 0.50 D.

- Where the refraction is one that the surgeon would usually adjust the treatment target by more than 0.50 D. (The manifest prescription is not always treated as the combination of the laser and the surgeon's technique has a unique combined effect on the outcome. Surgeons, therefore, develop a nomogram to enable them to adjust the treatment parameters to account for this effect.)

- Where the surgeon's nomogram indicates treating a different cylinder value to the aberrometer refraction. This is because the wavefront guided ablation program does not allow the surgeon to alter the cylinder treatment parameters.

- Where there are significant aberrations but corneal topography appears smooth, the origin of the aberration may not be corneal.

Wavefront guided ablation also removes more corneal tissue than conventional treatments and so is not always a suitable option for those patients with thin corneas.

Further reading

1. Smolek MK. The multimedia atlas of videokeratography. London: Butterworth-Heineman, 1999
2. Corbett MC, Rosen ES, O'Brart DPS. Corneal topography: principles and applications. Login Brothers Book Company, 1999
3. Naroo S. Refractive surgery: a guide to assessment and management. London: Butterworth-Heineman, 2004

References

1. Bethke W. Catching pathology: topography 101. Rev Ophthalmol 2004;11/04.
2. Touzeau O, Allouch C, Borderie V *et al*. Precision and reliability of Orbscan and ultrasonic pachymetry. J Fr Ophthalmol 2001;9:912–921.
3. Iskander NG, Anderson Penno E, Peters NT, Gimbel HV, Ferensowicz M. Accuracy of Orbscan pachymetry measurements and DHG ultrasound pachymetry in primary laser *in situ* keratomileusis and LASIK enhancement procedures. J Cataract Refract Surg 2001; 27:681–685.
4. Javaloy J, Vidal MT, Villada JR, Artola A, Alio JL. Comparison of four corneal pachymetry techniques in corneal refractive surgery. Refract Surg 2004;20:29–34.
5. Suzuki S, Oshika T, Oki K, Sakabe I, Iwase A, Amano S, Araie M. Corneal thickness measurements: scanning-slit corneal topography and noncontact specular microscopy versus ultrasonic pachymetry. Cataract Refract Surg 2003;29:1313–1318.
6. Partal AE, Manche EE. Diameters of topographic optical zone and programmed ablation zone for laser *in situ* keratomileusis for myopia. J Refract Surg 2003;19:528–533.
7. Kezirian GM. Rational patient selection for wavefront-guided LASIK. Rev Ophthalmol 2004;47–49.

Chapter **4**

Pre-operative assessment – eye examination

This chapter gives a detailed guide to carrying out the pre-operative assessment that is required to determine a patient's suitability for treatment. The treating surgeon will make the final decision regarding suitability and advise the patient regarding any risks specific to their case. Alternatives to LASIK and optometrist discharge is also discussed for when the patient is unsuitable for further consultation with the surgeon.

CONTENTS

INTRODUCTION

This chapter will look at the ocular examination and the further measurements required to determine a patient's suitability for treatment. It will also look at the optometrist's responsibility if the patient is discharged without treatment. A summary of alternative refractive procedures is also included at the end of this chapter which may be of use if the patient wishes to know more about an alternative to LASIK.

HISTORY AND SYMPTOMS

Absolute and relative contra-indications to surgery have been discussed in Chapter 2. Where the patient is taking a contra-indicated medication, it may be possible to treat them in the future once the medication has been ceased or changed to an alternative for several months. If the patient has a medical condition that is a relative contra-indication, the surgeon will need more information before making a final decision to treat the patient.

Diabetes

If the diabetes is well controlled and there are no signs of diabetic retinopathy, the surgeon may be prepared to operate on the patient. Further evidence of the status of the patient may be requested (*e.g.* the results of a haemoglobin AC1 test) and a report from the patient's diabetic physician.

Depression

In some cases, the surgeon may require a letter from the patient's GP stating that their condition is stable and that the patient is psychologically fit to undergo elective surgery. In many cases, these patients also have high expectations which, if not met, could disrupt their control of their depression. Therefore, it is imperative that these patients are counselled carefully about the potential risks and complications of surgery.

Dry eye

If a patient suffers from dry eye, their symptoms will be worse after treatment. Recovery could take several months. Where the dry eye is not severe and the patient is keen for treatment, punctum plugs can be inserted immediately after treatment to minimise discomfort.

Blepharitis

This will need to be treated prior to surgery. In most cases, lid hygiene measures are adequate as long as the patient is compliant. Where blepharitis is severe, topical or oral antibiotics may be required and referral to either the surgeon or the GP is required to obtain a prescription.

VISION ASSESSMENT

A full eye examination is carried out during the pre-operative assessment.

Refraction

The refraction result is compared to the patient's spectacles or most recent prescription. A difference of more than 0.50 D is significant and the patient will need to be rechecked again in 6–12 months' time. Suitability for treatment cannot be confirmed until the prescription is stable.

All hypermetropes will need a cycloplegic refraction. Where there is a large difference between the cycloplegic and the non-cycloplegic refraction, it may not be advisable to treat the maximum degree of hypermetropia as the patient may find it hard to adjust after treatment. In some cases, partial correction may be appropriate; in others, the patient may need to adapt to the cycloplegic result with spectacles or contact lenses before being considered for treatment.

In some cases, where a myope is suspected of over accommodating, a cycloplegic agent may also need to be instilled. The lowest myopic prescription found is then treated.

Best corrected visual acuity (BCVA)

If the patient has significant amblyopia or where the BCVA is less than 6/12, they will not be suitable for surgery. In cases where the amblyopia is mild, the patient needs to be counselled carefully about the potential risks and complications of surgery (see Chapter 5). Where the patient's BCVA is borderline, the surgeon may suggest treating one eye at a time with the amblyopic eye being treated first.

Binocular vision assessment

The binocular vision status of the patient should be assessed to identify patients who are unsuitable for treatment, or who are at increased risk of developing symptoms after treatment. The following is a list of potential problems:

- Patients that require prism to correct diplopia or decompensated heterophoria may still require spectacles after treatment.

- Moderate-to-high myopes have a significant degree of induced base in prism for near vision tasks with spectacles. If this is removed they may experience some eye strain after treatment until their eyes adapt. If the patient is exophoric or has convergence insufficiency, adaptation may not be possible and orthoptic exercises or prism correction may be required.

- If a pre-presbyopic myope habitually removes spectacles for near vision tasks, it could indicate that there are poor accommodative reserves. After treatment to correct the myopia, the patient will have to accommodate for reading. If the patient is unable to sustain this effort, then near vision spectacles may be required.

- If a myopic patient is esophoric for near and usually removes their spectacles for reading, the extra accommodation needed for near vision tasks after treatment will also increase convergence which may exacerbate a convergence excess esophoria, resulting in decompensation.

- Where the patient has a heterophoria that is poorly controlled, if the eyes are not perfectly binocularly balanced after surgery, it could result in a breaking down of the heterophoria into a heterotropia.

If there are any doubts about the patient's potential binocular vision after treatment, then contact lenses can be used to simulate the treatment correction. All problems associated with prism or accommodation will then be revealed except in the latter case, where treatment under or over correction is unintentional and, therefore, not predictable.

Ocular dominance testing

This is recorded as baseline data. This information will enable the surgeon to decide which eye should be undercorrected in the case of myopic presbyopes who want monovision. In other cases, where the corneal thickness is borderline for the patient's prescription, the patient may be happy to be slightly undercorrected in their non-dominant eye as it is unlikely to have a significant effect on the vision. This could mean the difference to being suitable or not suitable for LASIK.

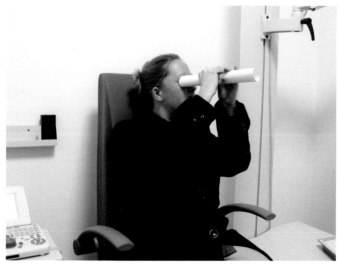

Figure 4.1   Ocular dominance testing

The simplest way to check ocular dominance is the 'paper telescope' test. A piece of paper is rolled up into a long tube and handed to the patient. The patient is then asked to hold it in both hands and to look through it as if it were a telescope. The patient will hold it up to their dominant eye (see Figure 4.1).

Another method is to ask the patient to fixate a distant target and then point directly at it. If the patient automatically closes one eye to fixate, then the dominant eye is usually the open eye. If both eyes are kept open, only the dominant eye will be in line with the target (Figure 4.2a). Covering each eye in turn will establish which eye is dominant. The example in Figure 4.2b shows a right dominant

(a)

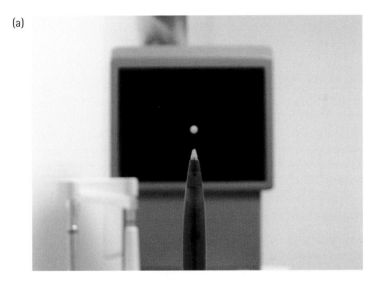

(b)

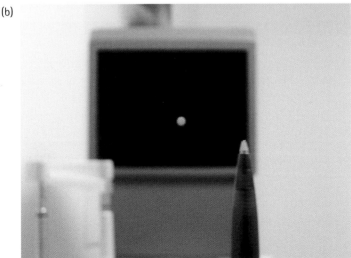

Figure 4.2 An alternative method of ocular dominance testing. (a) Target viewed through the dominant eye; (b) target viewed through the non-dominant eye

eye with the target being displaced when to the left when the right eye is closed. If there is displacement from the target in both eyes equally, there may be equal ocular dominance. Ocular dominance testing is not always consistent and it can also change between distance and near vision.

OCULAR EXAMINATION

If any of the following examinations reveal any potential contra-indications to surgery, the patient will need to be referred to the treating surgeon for an assessment before suitability for treatment can be confirmed. Ideally, this should be scheduled at least 24 hours prior to treatment day as indicated in The Royal College of Ophthalmologists' guidelines.

Anterior eye examination

The lids and lashes must be clear of any signs of blepharitis. The conjunctiva and sclera should also be quiet. The cornea should be checked for any corneal dystrophies or signs of previous herpetic activity. The anterior chamber should be examined and assessed prior to dilation. The lens is also checked for any signs of cataract, which if found, may alter the type of refractive surgery recommended to the patient.

Tear film assessment

The tear prism height will give an indication of tear volume; Figure 4.3 shows an adequate tear prism. Fluorescein has been used in this case to allow ease of observation but is not always necessary. Non-invasive tear break-up time will indicate

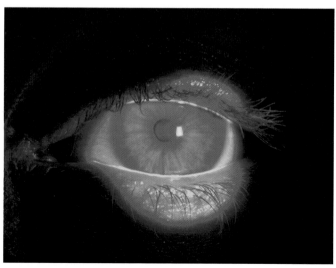

Figure 4.3   An indication of tear volume can be found by measuring the tear prism height

tear quality; this can be done by observing the tear film on a slit lamp or by observing keratometer mires (see Figure 4.4). In some cases, surgeons may prefer to use a Schirmer type test.

Dilated fundoscopy

The retina should be healthy and in particular, be checked for any signs of optic disc damage, retinopathy or peripheral retinal thinning dystrophies.

Tonometry

This measurement is required for baseline data purposes as it is likely to change after corneal surgery. The measurement can be taken with non-contact or contact tonometry or even both.

Endothelial cell analysis

This is an optional examination which can help to screen for corneal anomalies. If the endothelium has already been significantly compromised by contact lens overwear, it may alter the effectivity of the endothelial pump to resolve corneal oedema.

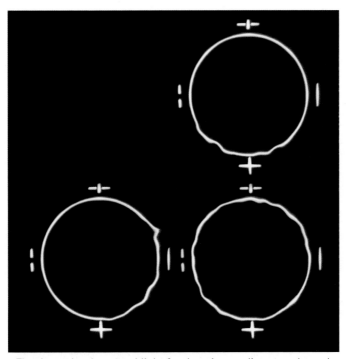

Figure 4.4   The time taken between blinks for the mires to distort as shown here is the tear break-up time which is an indicator of tear quality

PACHYMETRY

This measurement is an essential piece of pre-operative data which is used to calculate the residual stromal bed and ultimately determines whether or not the treatment can be carried out. Ultrasound pachymetry has been considered the gold standard but recent studies have shown that instruments such the Orbscan II which use a scanning slit also have good correlation on pre-operative corneas.[1-4]

The cornea is usually the thinnest at the centre and in keratoconus, at the apex of the cone. Therefore, when taking pachymetry measurements, it is best to check the topography for any potential corneal thinning dystrophies before relying on the central measurement. In the normal eye, the thinnest area is usually in the central area of the cornea. Thickness increases towards the periphery with the temporal cornea being thinner than the nasal.

Taking the measurement

1. Check that the probe head has been disinfected.
2. Instil a topical anaesthetic.
3. Place the tip of the probe so that it is normal to the cornea and make contact.
4. Most pachymeters beep when a reading has been taken.
5. Repeat the measurement to obtain an average of 3 readings.

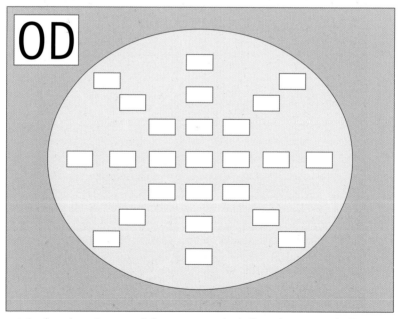

Figure 4.5 A pachymetry map of the cornea can be built up by systematically measuring different points of the cornea

6. Where topography indicates a localised area of steepening or flattening, carry out measurements in those areas.
7. It is then best to record these measurements as a pachymetry map (see Figure 4.5).

Suitability calculation

This can be done by the optometrist to rule out any obviously unsuitable patients before they have a final assessment with the surgeon. The ablation depth for each patient can be calculated using specific tables provided by the laser manufacturer which are based upon the Munnerlyn formula.[5]

$$\text{Depth of ablation} = (\text{Diameter of ablation})^2 \times (\text{Dioptres of correction})$$

Table 4.1 shows typical ablation depth per dioptre, and it can be seen that a greater treatment zone diameter requires a greater depth of ablation to achieve an equivalent amount of correction. Proprietary software results in different lasers ablating different amounts of tissue per dioptre of correction. The treatment zone is determined by the scotopic pupil measurement, and the dioptric power of the treatment is taken from the highest powered meridian of the patient's prescription. The ablation depth is read off the appropriate column and then subtracted from the lowest pachymetry measurement. The result indicates the total remaining corneal thickness. It is generally recognised by ophthalmologists that a minimum residual stromal bed thickness (RST) of 250 μm must remain under the flap after surgery. The flap thickness is usually set by the treating surgeon and depends upon the microkeratome being used. It can be between 110 and 180 μm.

The residual stromal bed must be ⩾ 250 μm
RST = Corneal thickness − (Ablation depth + Flap thickness)

Table 4.1 Ablation depth required per dioptre of correction for set treatment zones

	Required correction 6 mm treatment zone	Ablation depth (μm) 7 mm treatment zone
−1.00	12	16.3
−2.00	24	32.7
−3.00	36	49
−4.00	48	65.3
−5.00	60	81.7
−6.00	72	98
−7.00	84	114.3
−8.00	96	130.7

Example calculation
Scotopic pupil = 5.8 mm
Refractive error = −3.00/−3.00 × 180 (highest powered meridian
            = −6.00)
Pachymetry   = 540 µm

Assuming a treatment zone diameter of 6 mm
Flap thickness   = 160 µm
Ablation depth (from table) = 72 µm
RST   = 540 − 160 − 72 = 308 µm

This treatment can be safely carried out. It should be made clear to the patient that the final clinical suitability is decided upon by the treating surgeon who will also select the final surgical parameters. Any indication of suitability by the optometrist is for final assessment by the treating surgeon only and not for the treatment itself.

FINAL ASSESSMENT

If the patient is found to be suitable for treatment, they can then be booked in for surgery. The surgeon will need to meet the patient and check the notes to confirm suitability. The surgeon may also wish to check that all the patient's questions about treatment have been answered. This has usually been done on the day of treatment itself but recently, The Royal College of Ophthalmologists has produced guidelines indicating that this should be carried out at least 24 hours before treatment so that the patient has an adequate cooling-off period.

OPTOMETRIST DISCHARGE

If the patient is not suitable for treatment, other refractive surgery options may still be an option. A summary of these other options can be found at the end of this chapter. If the patient is not proceeding with treatment, the optometrist still has a duty of care to the patient to ensure that an examination to detect 'signs of injury, disease or abnormality in the eye' has been carried out according to *The Optician's Act (1989)*.[7] The purpose of the assessment is not a routine eye examination as in practice, but specific to determining suitability for treatment in the clinic. Therefore, it is not necessary to issue a prescription for spectacles. The patient should be informed that a routine eye examination should still be carried out by their own optometrist after the usual recall period. However, if any abnormality is found, it must be referred to the patient's GP.

OTHER REFRACTIVE SURGERY OPTIONS

Surface ablation

This refers to photorefractive keratectomy (PRK) and laser epithelial kerato-mileusis (LASEK). These two procedures are very similar and involve removing the epithelium before applying the laser. In PRK, the epithelium is removed using rotating abrasive brushes. In LASEK, ethanol is applied for up to 30 s to loosen the epithelium before it is peeled back. It can then be replaced after treatment, whereas in PRK, the epithelium needs to regenerate completely. At the end of the LASEK procedure, a bandage contact lens is applied to the eye which helps to keep the epithelium in place. Epi-LASIK (epipolis laser in situ keratomileusis) is an alternative method of lifting the epithelial flap mechanically using a blunt oscillating blade rather than an alcohol solution. It is still a relatively new technique and few studies have been performed to date.[8]

Surface ablation surgery is not subject to the same risks as LASIK where a flap is cut using a microkeratome, but the risk of haze and regression is greater in larger corrections. It is also possible for the epithelial flap to become detached during treatment, so the surgeon may attempt LASEK, but actually carry out PRK. This method of treatment is suitable for mild-to-moderate myopes whose corneas are thin, for which LASIK may not be possible. It may also be more suitable than LASIK for those patients who are at high risk of ocular trauma in their occupation or hobbies. Early postoperative discomfort is greater with surface treatments, but final visual outcome is similar to that of LASIK.

Some studies have indicated that the benefits of the LASEK 'epi-flap' were faster healing, reduced risk of haze and less postoperative pain than with PRK.[9] Other studies have not supported this,[10] with one study stating 'no additional clinical benefit is seen from the LASEK procedure relative to the PRK procedure'.[11] It is generally accepted that more studies are needed to understand the potential benefits of LASEK.[12] The LASEK technique is discussed in more detail in Chapter 10.

Radial keratotomy

Radial incisions which may involve up to 90% of the corneal thickness are arranged in a concentric pattern around a central optic zone. The refractive effect is controlled by the number and depth of incisions, as well as the size of the central clear zone. The effect will depend upon the age of the patient. It can be used to correct mild degrees of myopia, and is now used more as secondary technique to correct residual myopia after other surgical procedures.

A variation of this is astigmatic keratotomy, where an incision is made perpendicular to the axis of the steepest meridian. This has the effect of flattening that meridian and correcting the astigmatism. The degree of flattening depends upon the length, depth and position of the incision. It can be used to correct up to 4.00 D of astigmatism.

Clear lens extraction and intraocular lens (IOL) implant

This procedure is essentially the same as modern cataract surgery except that the lens is removed before opacification has occurred. The IOL implant that is used to replace the natural lens is calculated to correct the refractive error of the patient. Toric IOLs are also being used by some surgeons, although the outcome for correcting corneal astigmatism is less predictable. Any residual prescription can be treated with LASIK or surface ablation. If there is any astigmatic error, it could also be treated with astigmatic keratotomy.

This procedure is particularly suitable for presbyopes who may have early lens opacities and for those patients whose refractive error is too great to be corrected safely with LASIK or surface ablation. Although cataract extraction and the insertion of IOLs is a relatively common procedure, it is not without risk and this should be discussed with the treating surgeon. The main risks associated with this type of surgery are infection. The risk of retinal detachment also increases after surgery.

The loss of accommodation makes this procedure unsuitable for young patients and although multifocal implants are available, they do not consistently provide good near vision for all patients. Implants that simulate accommodation are also emerging and in time, they may remove this barrier to lens extraction in pre-presbyopic patients.

Phakic intraocular lens implant

This procedure for myopia is carried out when the patient's own crystalline lens needs to be preserved. The lens can be placed in the anterior chamber, fixed to the iris or in the posterior chamber. This procedure is less popular now due to the advances made in alternative techniques.

Implantable contact lens (ICL)

This is a reversible procedure which allows the correction of high degrees of myopia and, in some cases, hypermetropia. It is primarily used when corneal surgery is not suitable and where accommodation needs to be preserved. The ICL is inserted through a small sutureless incision into the posterior chamber but does not touch the crystalline lens. Potential complications include endothelial or lens trauma, and lens decentration. Peripheral iridectomy is also required with this procedure to prevent pupil block glaucoma. Visual complications include glare, haloes and ghosting when the pupil dilates in scotopic conditions due to the edge of the ICL falling within the pupillary area.

Intrastromal corneal ring segments (ICRS)

These are curved polymethylmethacrylate corneal implants that extend 150° of arc that are placed at a depth of 66% of the corneal thickness in the peripheral cornea. The distension in the periphery causes a flattening of the central cornea

Table 4.2   Summary of alternative refractive surgery procedures

Procedure	Treatment range	Accommo-dation preserved	Reversible	Risks specific to treatment	Risks that apply to all treatments
Surface ablation (PRK/LASEK)	+1.00 to −4.00 D	Yes	No	Haze Regression	Infection
Radial keratotomy	Up to −6.00 D	Yes	No	Micro-perforation Progressive hypermetropia Endothelial cell loss Limited predictability Variable vision	Inflammation Under/over correction
Phakic IOL Intraocular contact lenses	Manufacturer's availability	Yes	Yes	Endothelial cell loss Crystalline lens trauma Lens opacities	Induced astigmatism
Aphakic IOL	Manufacturer's availability	No	No	Endothelial cell loss Increased risk of retinal detachment	Irregular astigmatism
Intrastromal corneal ring segments	−1.00 to −3.00 D	Yes	Yes	Stromal deposits Focusing difficulties Discomfort	Glare, haloes, ghosting

and a subsequent reduction in myopia. The reduction depends upon the thickness of the implant and can correct between 1.00 and 4.00 D of spherical myopia. Sutures are not required and the procedure is also reversible as no corneal tissue is removed. The procedure is very safe and complications, although rare, include induced astigmatism, vascular ingrowth, and peripheral stromal deposits. Visual complications include glare, focusing difficulty and discomfort. This technique can also be used to manage keratoconus.

A summary of the main features of these techniques is presented in Table 4.2.

References

1. Touzeau O, Allouch C, Borderie V, Ameline B, Chastang P, Bouzegaou F, Laroche L. Precision and reliability of Orbscan and ultrasonic pachymetry. J Fr Ophtalmol 2001;24:912–921.

2. Iskander NG, Anderson Penno E, Peters NT, Gimbel HV, Ferensowicz M. Accuracy of Orbscan pachymetry measurements and DHG ultrasound pachymetry in primary laser *in situ* keratomileusis and LASIK enhancement procedures. J Cataract Refract Surg 2001;27:681–685.

3. Javaloy J, Vidal MT, Villada JR, Artola A, Alio JL. Comparison of four corneal pachymetry techniques in corneal refractive surgery. J Refract Surg 2004;20:29–34.

4. Suzuki S, Oshika T, Oki K, Sakabe I, Iwase A, Amano S, Araie M. Corneal thickness measurements: scanning-slit corneal topography and noncontact specular microscopy versus ultrasonic pachymetry. J Cataract Refract Surg 2003;29:1313–1318.

5. Munnerlyn CR, Koons SJ, Marshall J. Photorefractive keratectomy: a technique for laser refractive surgery. J Cataract Refract Surg 14:46–52.

6. The Royal College of Ophthalmologists. Standards for laser refractive surgery. London: The Royal College of Ophthalmologists, 2003.

7. The Sight Testing (examination and prescribing) (No. 2) Regulations (1989).

8. Pallikaris IG, Katsanevaki VJ, Kalyvianaki MI, Naoumidi II. Advances in subepithelial excimer refractive surgery techniques: Epi-LASIK. Curr Opin Ophthalmol 2003;14:207–212.

9. Camellin M. Laser epithelial keratomileusis for myopia. J Refract Surg 2003;19:666–670.

10. Litwak S, Zadok D, Garcia-de Quevedo V, Robledo N, Chayet AS. Assisted subepithelial keratectomy versus photorefractive keratectomy for the correction of myopia. A prospective comparative study. J Cataract Refract Surg 2002;28:1330–1333.

11. Pirouzian A, Thornton JA, Ngo S. A randomized prospective clinical trial comparing laser subepithelial keratomileusis and photorefractive keratectomy. Arch Ophthalmol 2004;122:11–16.

12. Ambrosio Jr R, Wilson S. LASIK vs LASEK vs PRK: advantages and indications. Semin Ophthalmol 2003;18:2–10.

Chapter 5

Pre-operative assessment – patient counselling

OVERVIEW

Informed consent is a requirement before all surgical procedures. Before a consent form can be signed, it is necessary that the patient fully understands the treatment that they are receiving. The patient must know the benefits of treatment as well as the alternative methods of correcting their vision. It is imperative that they fully understand the potential risks and complications of the procedure as well as the management and outcomes of such incidences. The information in this chapter is not necessarily what the patient needs to be told, but will provide the background information needed by the optometrist to counsel the patient.

CONTENTS

INTRODUCTION

Once the patient has been determined to be clinically suitable for treatment, it is essential to ensure that the limitations of surgery are understood and that the risks associated with LASIK are explained. The majority of patients are happy with the outcome of their surgery but all surgery involves some risk of complications and the outcome may not satisfy the patient's expectations. These expectations will have arisen from the knowledge of friends that have undergone treatment and from the marketing campaigns of laser refractive surgery providers.

Competition for patients between the providers of laser refractive surgery has led to prominent publicity campaigns often endorsed by celebrities from both the fashion and sporting worlds. Booklets and videos have been produced by clinics to give patients more information about their treatment and the benefits of choosing that individual clinic. The marketing strategy of clinics has inevitably created high public expectations. Patients believe the surgery to be simple and risk free, with immediate results. The Advertising Standards Agency is responsible for investigating complaints about misrepresentation in advertising and has helped to keep the marketing of LASIK fair and accurate. The GOC and the GMC also have regulations relating to the marketing of services which also serve to protect the public.

The public desire for an easy solution to their eyesight problems cannot be underestimated and it is likely that some patients will take more risk to gain a more convenient recovery with less pain. However, when considering surgery, the risks and benefits of treatment must be discussed in detail with the patient before proceeding.

Patients vary a great deal in the amount of knowledge they have about LASIK. Some patients know absolutely nothing and others attend for consultation armed with information gleaned from several sources such as the internet. Patients have an increasing amount of information available to them and there are some very good information sites for patients considering treatment, for example, <www.cycsurgcrycducation.com> cstablishcd by thc Amcrican Association of Cataract and Refractive Surgeons. Patients are able to research into current surgical techniques, clinics and even surgeons using the internet. However, there are also several sites dedicated to 'disasters'. Therefore, when the optometrist or surgeon discusses surgery, the attitude of the patient needs to be considered so that their concerns are answered appropriately. Some patients also find it useful to have a partner or friend with them during this part of the consultation as they can feel overwhelmed by all the information and forget some of it.

MANAGING PATIENT EXPECTATIONS

Patients are asked what they expect their vision to be like after LASIK. They often give the following typical answers:

- 'I expect the vision to be the same as or better than in my contact lenses'

- 'I want to be able to drive and play sports without spectacles or contact lenses'
- 'I hope to be able to manage without spectacles most of the time'

The key words in these answers are 'expect', 'want' and 'hope'. The way the patient expresses their expectation often indicates their knowledge of the limitations of treatment and the manner in which they answer can indicate whether or not they are likely to be amenable to compromise if necessary.

Some patients are very specific and very firm about their high expectations. These patients are unlikely to be satisfied with anything other than a perfect result and so they need to be informed in no uncertain terms that this cannot be guaranteed. Where the patient 'expects' perfect vision, it is important first of all to determine exactly what they think is 'perfect' vision. For some patients perfect means their best corrected acuity, for others it means better. Other patients that expect 6/6 vision do not often know what it means and showing the difference between that and the equivalent driving standard is often enough to moderate their expectations. Explaining to the patient that they do not need 6/6 vision to gain functional independence from spectacles or contact lenses can be the first step in making their expectations realistic.

Where patients express a 'want' they are usually fairly realistic but are uncertain what the limitations of the treatment are and need more information on what is a realistic expectation. The most informed patients tend to be less specific with their expectations and 'hope' for good vision which they associate with being able to do certain tasks.

DISPELLING THE MYTHS

This section describes the some of the misconceptions about laser refractive surgery and some suggested explanations of the real situation to patients.

- **Myth** – LASIK will correct my vision to 20/20 without spectacles or contact lenses.

- **Fact** – Patients are not usually aware that 20/20 is a clinical measurement rather than a concept of perfect vision. Patients are also more familiar with the term '20/20' that is still used in some countries rather than the metric equivalent of 6/6. The treatment aims for a similar level of vision to that achieved with spectacles or contact lenses. This may well be 6/6 or better. However, each patient responds differently to treatment and regression is possible as the cornea heals. Therefore, although the vision may be good after treatment, it may not be the same as with spectacles or equivalent to 6/6. In some cases, the acuity may not be the same in each eye and 6/6 may only be reached binocularly.

- **Myth** – LASIK will give me 'perfect' vision.

- **Fact** – The vision after treatment is excellent in the majority of cases with some patients seeing 6/45 or better. However, visual acuity is only a single clinical measurement and does not take into account all the features of vision that make it perfect. The quality of vision can be altered after treatment due to changes in corneal transparency and the presence of debris. Some patients also notice a decrease in their ability to see at night which recovers after 6 months in most cases when the flap has completely settled.

> **Hint** – It often helps to show the patient the 6/6 line and to compare this to their best corrected vision. This usually gives them an appreciation of how well their vision is corrected with spectacles, especially when compared with the Snellen equivalent for legal driving.

- **Myth** – An outcome of less than 20/20 is an unsatisfactory result.
- **Fact** – Not all patients achieve 20/20 vision after treatment, yet most are still satisfied with the result.[1] A satisfactory result depends on whether the patient can see well enough to do the visual tasks they require without the help of spectacles. This does not necessarily mean 20/20 vision. The equivalent standard for driving is much less demanding and some patients, especially those with high prescriptions will be satisfied if they only have to wear spectacles for driving instead of all the time.

> **Tip** – A comparison between unaided vision and corrected acuity will demonstrate the aim of the treatment to the patient. Blurring induced by +0.50 will also demonstrate that a zero prescription is not needed for functional independence from spectacles.

- **Myth** – After LASIK, I will never need spectacles ever again.
- **Fact** – Where possible, the treatment aims to provide visual independence from corrective lenses but the eyes may continue to change throughout life and progression of myopia could still occur even after full correction. There is also a small risk of under or overcorrection with LASIK, so spectacles may still be required for some visual tasks if retreatment cannot be undertaken. As the ageing process continues, the eyes will not be able to focus at all distances, therefore spectacles for near vision tasks will be required after the age of 40–45 years.
- **Myth** – Wavefront treatment will give me 'super' vision and can guarantee a good visual result.
- **Fact** – Wavefront technology allows the aberrations of the eye to be measured before treatment. The laser can then be configured to correct these aberrations. However, good results are not always guaranteed as corneal aberrations do not remain constant from before to after treatment.
- **Myth** – I will definitely need reading glasses after LASIK.

- **Fact** – Some presbyopic patients are aware that although refractive error can be corrected by LASIK, presbyopia cannot be corrected in this manner. This is true. However, it may be possible to provide a reading correction by monovision. This is achieved in myopes by the deliberate undercorrection of the less dominant eye to leave it myopic. Where the patient is hypermetropic, an overcorrection is a possibility, but is rarely done as it could mean worsening the vision in an eye that can normally see reasonably well in the distance. The hypermetropic presbyope can still expect some improvement in their near vision after treatment, but not to the degree of a near add equivalent.

- **Myth** – My near vision is very good and I only need LASIK to correct my poor distance vision.

- **Fact** – Presbyopic myopes are often unaware that correcting their myopia with LASIK reveals the effects of presbyopia (*i.e.* blurred near vision). Some patients are quite put out by that fact and are, therefore, unlikely to be suitable candidates for full correction. For example, if a patient is a VDU worker and does not need their spectacles for work and only puts them on to drive home and watch TV, then it is arguable as to whether they actually need treatment at all as they may end up wearing spectacles more often after treatment if their myopia is corrected. In other cases, patients may feel as if they are only swapping one pair of spectacles for another. In these cases, it is up to the patient to decide whether the near or distance vision is their priority. Pre-presbyopic myopes must also be made aware that the near vision will be different once they have been corrected to near emmetropia.

> **Tip** – Demonstrating the effect of full distance correction with contact lenses and instructing the patient to look at different targets at various distances (especially looking at themselves in the mirror!) can help them to understand what to expect after treatment. This can then be followed with a monovision demonstration if necessary.

- **Myth** – If my prescription keeps changing I can have more treatment in the future.

- **Fact** – Where the vision is not satisfactory after LASIK, further treatment may be possible once the cornea has settled down. Any further treatment is only possible if there is adequate corneal tissue available to ablate. If myopia progresses several years after treatment, the possibility of re-treatment is still governed by the available corneal tissue. Treatment is delayed until the patient's prescription is stable, as relying on an indefinite number of treatments to keep correcting the vision is not practical.

- **Myth** – It is safer for my eyes if I have one eye treated at a time.

- **Fact** – Simultaneous bilateral LASIK is as safe and effective as sequential surgery.[2] If each eye is treated with a separate set of equipment, there is no increased risk to the second eye.

- **Myth** – The procedure is painless.

- **Fact** – The eyelids must be held apart by a speculum and a suction ring is placed onto the conjunctiva. This may require some manoeuvring which the patient may find uncomfortable. A local anaesthetic is used on the cornea so the procedure is painless; however, when the anaesthetic wears off, the patient may feel some discomfort ranging from grittyness to mild pain.

VISION AFTER TREATMENT

By this stage, the patient should have realistic expectations of the potential visual outcome. The next step is to prepare the patient for what their vision will be like after treatment, as many of them will feel much less anxious if they know what to expect.

Visual recovery

All patients are advised to go home and rest after treatment and to avoid visually stressful tasks. Although the vision will seem quite hazy, it will be much clearer the next day and the patient will be able to return to work. However, visual recovery can vary and some patients may find their vision improves more slowly over a few days. Patients are advised not to drive until after their first aftercare when their vision will be checked.

Presbyopia

Presbyopic myopes who are opting for full correction are warned that they will lose their unaided near vision. They will need to become accustomed to doing some tasks with blurred vision (*e.g.* applying makeup or shaving). If the patient is accustomed to removing spectacles for near work, then they will need to put a pair on after treatment instead. The vision can take several weeks to stabilize, so the patient is often advised to use ready readers temporarily after treatment until a pair of reading spectacles can be prescribed accurately.

Contact lenses simulation   If the patient remains unsure about whether to opt for full correction or monovision, then it is worth simulating the effect with disposable contact lenses. If this cannot be done at the clinic, it may mean referring the patient back to their optometrist or contact lens optician. With contact lenses fitted to emulate the correction, presbyopic myopes will be able to experience the blurring of their near vision. If this is unacceptable then monovision can be trialled.

Monovision   Unless patients have tried monovision in contact lenses already, they are normally reluctant to take an option that sounds unnatural to them. Monovision has been shown to be successful with LASIK[3,4] and where the patient is in doubt about being able to cope, a contact lens simulation is invaluable. Some surgeons do not provide the full reading add to the near vision eye if it is greater than 1.5 D as the myopic blur may confuse the clear image of the other eye. Even where the full add is not provided, patients tend to prefer some reading add to none at all as it still provides some independence from reading spectacles. In some cases, where the degree of myopia is similar to the reading add, the patient may opt to have only their dominant eye corrected.

RISKS AND COMPLICATIONS

All surgical procedures involve some risk and the patient can be lulled into a false sense of security by the ready availability of treatment in private clinics and hospitals. It is important to ensure that the patient understands the potential risks so that they can weigh up the benefits of having treatment with the risk of experiencing complications. It is essential to discuss these issues with the patient before they are asked to read and sign a consent form. This next section is a brief description of the potential complications to help the optometrist in counselling the patient. These complications and their management will be discussed in more detail in later chapters.

> **Tip** – The patient will hear a great deal of information and must understand it before they commit to having surgery. Therefore, it is helpful if they bring someone with them into this part of the consultation to help them remember the points discussed.

LASIK is not an intraocular procedure, so the risk of sight-threatening complications is low. The first question a patient wants to ask is: 'can I go blind with this treatment?'. At the time of writing, there were no reported cases of complete visual loss. However, there are other milder complications that the patient must be informed of. They can be divided into four main categories.

Infection or inflammation

Following treatment, the eye is more vulnerable to microbial attack. These potentially sight-threatening complications are unlikely as prophylactic antimicrobials are given to the patient to help prevent infection. Patient compliance is essential here and cannot be stressed heavily enough. There is also a risk of inflammation after treatment. This is controlled by the use of topical steroids. The patient is reviewed within 3 days of treatment, where the recovery progress of the corneas is checked. If the drug regimen is found to be inadequate, then the drug, dose or frequency can be amended appropriately. The patient is then followed up more closely until the infection or inflammation has been resolved.

Diffuse lamellar keratitis (DLK) is an inflammatory condition which has been found exclusively after LASIK. It has very little or no effect on the final visual outcome if detected and treated at an early stage. As the complication can be asymptomatic at its early stages, adherence to the aftercare schedule is imperative. Manifestation is usually within 48–72 hours but later onset has been reported.[5]

Flap complications

The incidence of microkeratome flap complications is low with one study quoting 2.27%,[6] another recent study carried out in the US looked at procedures carried out with a Hansatome microkeratome of which 46 out of 28 201 (0.16%) had a complication.[7] On the other hand, the same study found a complication rate of 6.38% with another microkeratome. This latter complication incidence seems to be an exception rather than the rule. It is also generally accepted that the complication rate decreases very rapidly upon the surgeon gaining experience.[8,9]

A failed flap can occur for several reasons. For example:

- Inadequate suction obtained prior the cutting of the flap.
- The patient trying to squeeze their eyes as the microkeratome passes over the cornea.
- Inadequate assembly of the microkeratome.
- Epithelium has a predisposition to poor adhesion or abrasion.

There are several types of flap complications:

- **Buttonhole flap** – a small tear or cut in the central region of the flap.
- **Free cap** – incision which completely removes the flap.
- **Incomplete flap** – where the mircokeratome does not complete the cutting procedure.
- **Thin flap** – where the flap created is too thin to continue with treatment without risking further complications.
- **Irregular/small flaps** – where the flap is malformed and treatment cannot be continued.
- **Epithelial abrasions** – usually caused as the microkeratome passes across the cornea. Some corneas have a pre-disposition to abrasions which has been linked to race and age in studies.

In many cases, surgery is aborted. Although classed as a complication, it does not usually have a long-term effect as the cornea returns to its normal refractive status and a second treatment can be attempted after the appropriate recovery period (approximately 3 months). The patient must be made aware that the final visual outcome of their treatment is unlikely to be affected.[8]

Flap displacement   Once the flap is placed back onto the stromal bed, it is kept in place by the suction action created by the endothelial pump. As the epithelium regenerates, it grows over the flap edge which further increases flap adherence. Until this latter stage begins to occur, the flap is very easily displaced causing striae and wrinkles in the flap. Therefore, the patient is given protective eye shields to wear after treatment to prevent eye rubbing. After the initial 48 hours, the flap is reasonably secure but it can still be displaced by significant rubbing for up to 4 weeks after treatment.[10] Long term, the flap can be displaced by severe ocular trauma and this has been documented in ophthalmic literature.[11,12] Therefore, where a patient is likely to be in frequent high-risk situations in the future (*e.g.* martial arts, contact sports), they should be advised of this risk accordingly. Visual recovery is usually successful following flap repositioning.[13] The appropriate use of safety eye wear in high risk situations (*e.g.* contact sports) is advisable for all patients, not just those who have had LASIK.

Laser complications

Significantly decentred ablations are less likely due to advances made in eye tracking technology. The surgeon also ensures by means of a video camera that centration is maintained during ablation. If misalignment occurs, the laser firing can be stopped and restarted if necessary.

Visual aberrations are another complication associated with corneal surgery. Central islands can occur due to the non-uniform ablation of the cornea which may cause some aberrations. This is prevented by ensuring that fluid does not collect on the stromal bed during ablation. Uneven hydration of the cornea during treatment can also create an irregular surface on stromal bed which may cause some aberrations in the vision. This is usually avoided by drying the stromal surface prior to ablation. In many cases, the aberrations resolve spontaneously as the cornea settles.[14] If still present after 6 months, many aberrations can be treated with further customised ablation.[15]

Visual complications

Loss of best corrected visual acuity (BCVA)   It is important to explain to all patients what the definition of BCVA is, so that they can fully understand the risks involved. All patients are informed of the possibility of a loss in BCVA of one or two lines. This is more likely with high refractive errors, especially high hypermetropia due to absence of magnification through spectacles. A loss in BCVA can also be caused by induced aberrations such as ghosting (see Figure 5.1), the risk is minimised by good surgical technique during laser ablation and in the replacing of the flap after treatment. It is important to stress to those patients whose BCVA pre-operatively is 6/7.5 or less that if BCVA is reduced by more than 2 lines, their vision may not be adequate for legal driving. For this reason, patients with an amblyopic eye which cannot see better than 6/12 are often refused treatment.

Under/over correction   This is defined as when the treatment does not provide the desired correction of the refractive error and is usually apparent at the first aftercare if there are no other complications to affect the vision. The risk of significant undercorrection increases with refractive error.[16] The actual correction does not rely on just the correct information being entered onto the laser computer by the laser operator, but the following factors can also influence the outcome.

- Incorrect pre-operative refractive measurement.
- Hydration of the cornea during ablation.
- Humidity and temperature of operating theatre (usually monitored and kept constant).

The treatment is based upon the average healing properties of the cornea, but small variations will occur between individuals. The latter two factors are accounted for by the treating surgeon with the use of a purpose-calculated algorithm which is specific for each combination of surgeon and laser. Any residual or induced prescription can be treated at later date provided that the corneal thickness is adequate.

Regression   Some patients may respond very well to treatment and reach the required level of vision after initial recovery. However, the surgical result can be lessened after an initial period of stability due to the biomechanical response of the cornea as it heals. The remaining prescription can usually be retreated as long

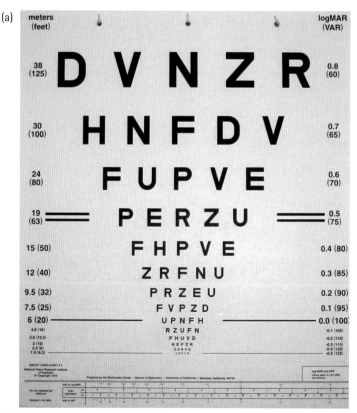

Figure 5.1(a)   A Bailey-Lovie chart viewed without aberrations (*continued on next page*)

(b)

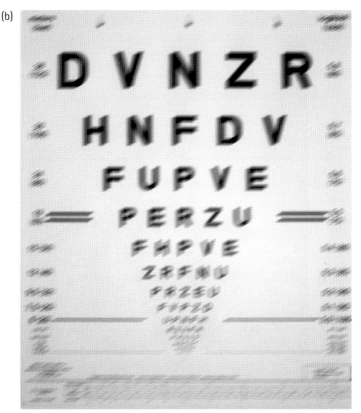

Figure 5.1   (b) The effect of ghosting with a reduction in visual acuity and quality (*continued from previous page*)

as the corneal parameters are still suitable. Where patients have a high pre-operative prescription, the potential eligibility for further treatment will need to be discussed carefully before consenting to the first procedure.

Ectasia   This is a rare complication caused by the lowering of the strength and tension in the corneal lamellae which results in a significant increase in the curvature of the posterior and anterior corneal surfaces. It is associated with a stromal bed thickness of less than 250 µm and corneal thinning dystophies.[17] The risk of ectasia is minimised by ensuring that the stromal bed remaining after ablation is at least 250 µm deep.

Glare, haloes and starburst   Treatment disrupts the corneal transparency which can result in glare effects. These include:

- **Discomfort glare** – increased sensitivity to bright conditions.
- **Disability glare** – also called veiling glare with causes the vision to feel slightly hazy in bright conditions. Figure 5.2 shows a city scene with neon lights and

(a)

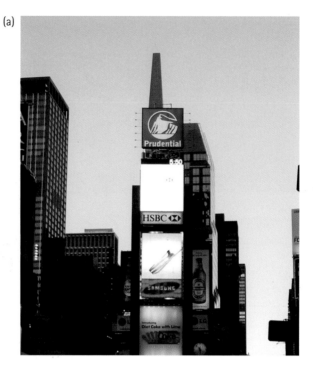

(b)

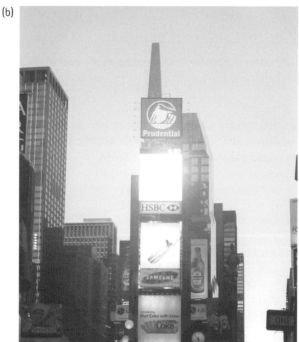

Figure 5.2 (a) A city scene as it appears to a person with normal vision; (b) The glare effectively 'veils' the scene thus reducing the saturation of colours and reducing contrast

it can be seen that the general glare reduces the contrast of the whole scene and is more noticeable around very bright light sources.

- **Haloes** – light sources against a dark background appear to have a halo of light around them (see Figure 5.3).
- **Starburst** – bright light sources appear to have darts of light coming out of them. Figure 5.4 is a diagrammatic representation of starburst on a pair of car headlights seen under scotopic conditions.

Patients will be particularly aware of these effects at night during the first few days after treatment. The patient may also feel particularly photophobic for the first 24 hours after treatment. In most cases, the symptoms improve significantly within a few days and then a more gradual improvement occurs for up to 6 months.

Reduced contrast sensitivity   After treatment, the patient may suffer a temporary decrease in contrast sensitivity which the patient notices as reduced night vision. This is well documented in studies and has also been shown to return to pre-operative levels after 3 months.[18,19] Patients may also notice this when they are trying carry out visual tasks that have poor contrast (*e.g.* reading small print on coloured backgrounds). Reduced contrast can be demonstrated by using the Pelli-Robson contrast sensitivity chart or the reduced contrast Bailey-Lovie chart (see Figure 5.5).

> **Hint** – If reduced contrast charts are not available, turning the background illumination off on an illuminated Snellen chart or introducing a tinted lens sample will also do. An 85% transmission factor will give a subtle change to contrast sensitivity or using the polarising filters from the Mallett test on a normal Snellen chart will demonstrate a more obvious change.

Dry eye

Most patients notice dry eye symptoms after treatment due to a disruption of the corneal nerves which control tear production resulting in a lower tear volume. In some cases, tear disruption has been reported for up to 9 months.[20] This is resolved by the use of ocular lubricants postoperatively until symptoms subside. This is usually between 1 and 6 months and is highly variable from one individual to the next.

> **Hint** – Telling the patient that dry eye feels like a soft contact lens that has been worn for too long is a good way of conveying the potential symptoms of grittiness and fluctuating vision.

CONSENT FORM

Once the potential complications have been explained, the patient should be given a copy of the consent form to take home and read. The Royal College of

(a)

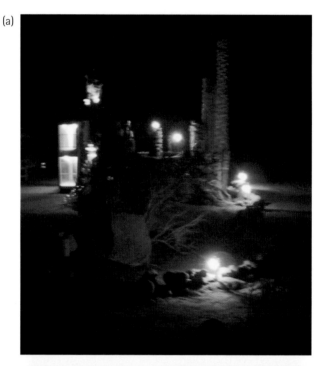

(b)

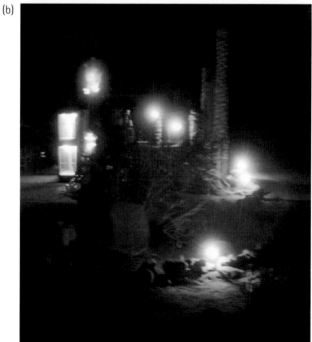

Figure 5.3   (a) The appearance of lights at night; (b) At night, haloes may be seen around the light sources

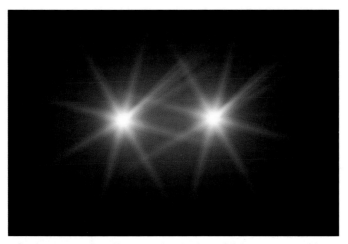

Figure 5.4 Starburst can also affect a patient's view of light sources and it more noticeable at night

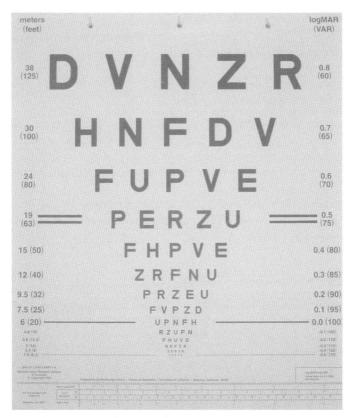

Figure 5.5 A reduced contrast Bailey-Lovie chart

Ophthalmologists recommends that this should be at least 24 hours before treatment. It should be read prior to treatment day to ensure that the patient has had time to understand fully the nature of the consent form and to ask any further questions. If the patient is only given the consent form just before they have treatment, when they are likely to be highly nervous, it is more likely to scare them and to delay or cancel treatment.

INSTRUCTIONS FOR TREATMENT DAY

If the patient decides to go ahead with treatment, they are usually given a written list of instructions to adhere to prior to arriving at the clinic for treatment. This may include the following:

- Make sure you have left your contact lenses out for the required period before treatment day.
- Make sure you have read your consent form before arriving at the clinic.
- Come accompanied to the clinic as your vision will be hazy after treatment for several hours and you will not be able to drive home.
- Bring sunglasses to wear after treatment as your eyes will be sensitive to light after treatment.
- Do not wear any makeup, perfume or aftershave on the day of treatment.
- Do not return to work on the treatment day as you need to rest and allow your eyes to recover.
- Ensure that you have made arrangements to come back to the clinic for your first aftercare within 4 days of treatment.

Patients often find that they are given so much information that they cannot make a decision immediately on whether to have treatment or not. Even when patients are eager to have treatment, the Royal College of Ophthalmologists' guidelines state that a minimum cooling-off period of overnight is required. This is good practice as it allows the patient to reflect on the information given and to ensure that they understand all the implications of signing the consent form. The patient should be given a contact telephone number just in case they think of any other questions after they have left.

References

1. Bailey MD, Mitchell GL, Dhaliwal DK *et al.* Patient satisfaction and visual symptoms after laser *in situ* keratomileusis. Ophthalmology 2003;110:1371–1378.
2. Gimbel HV, van Westenbrugge JA, Penno EE *et al.* Simultaneous bilateral laser *in situ* keratomileusis: safety and efficacy. Ophthalmology 1999;106:1461–1467; discussion 1467–1468.
3. Goldberg DB. Laser *in situ* keratomileusis monovision. J Cataract Refract Surg 2001;27:1449–1455.
4. Jain S, Ou R, Azar DT. Monovision outcomes in presbyopic individuals after refractive surgery. Ophthalmology 2001;108:1430–1433.

5. Asano-Kato N, Toda I, Tsubota K. Severe late-onset recurrent epithelial erosion with diffuse lamellar keratitis after laser *in situ* keratomileusis. J Cataract Refract Surg 2003;29:2019–2021.

6. Lui MM, Silas MA, Fugishima H. Complications of photorefractive keratectomy and laser *in situ* keratomileusis. J Cataract Refract Surg 2003;19(2 Suppl):S247–S249.

7. Jacobs JM, Taravella MJ. Incidence of intraoperative flap complications in laser *in situ* keratomileusis. J Cataract Refract Surg 2002;28:23–28.

8. Tham VM, Maloney RK. Microkeratome complications of laser *in situ* keratomileusis. Ophthalmology 2000;107:920–924.

9. Stulting RD, Carr JD, Thompson KP *et al.* Complications of laser *in situ* keratomileusis for the correction of myopia. Ophthalmology 1999;106:13–20.

10. Sridhar MS, Rapuano CJ, Cohen EJ. Accidental self-removal of a flap – a rare complication of laser *in situ* keratomileusis surgery. Am J Ophthalmol 2001;132: 780–782.

11. Lemley HL, Chodosh J, Wolf TC *et al.* Partial dislocation of laser *in situ* keratomileusis flap by air bag injury. J Refract Surg 2000;16:373–374.

12. Tumbocon JA, Paul R, Slomovic A *et al.* Late traumatic displacement of laser *in situ* keratomileusis flaps. Cornea 2003;22:66–69.

13. Aldave AJ, Hollander DA, Abbott RL. Late-onset traumatic flap dislocation and diffuse lamellar inflammation after laser *in situ* keratomileusis. Cornea 2002;21:604–607.

14. Lee JS, Joo CK. Central islands after LASIK detected by corneal topography. Korean J Ophthalmol 2001;15:8–14.

15. Manche EE, Maloney RK, Smith RJ. Treatment of topographic central islands following refractive surgery. J Cataract Refract Surg 1998;24:464–470.

16. Hersh PS, Fry KL, Bishop DS. Incidence and associations of retreatment after LASIK. Ophthalmology 2003;110:748–754.

17. Schmitt-Bernard CF, Lesage C, Arnaud B. Keratectasia induced by laser *in situ* keratomileusis in keratoconus. J Refract Surg 2000;16:368–370.

18. Mutyala S, McDonald MB, Scheinblum KA *et al.* Contrast sensitivity evaluation after laser *in situ* keratomileusis. Ophthalmology 2000;107:1864–1867.

19. Perez-Santonja JJ, Sakla HF, Alio JL. Contrast sensitivity after laser *in situ* keratomileusis. J Cataract Refract Surg 1998;24:183–189.

20. Benitez-del-Castillo JM, del Rio T, Iradier T *et al.* Decrease in tear secretion and corneal sensitivity after laser *in situ* keratomileusis. Cornea 2001;20:30–32.

Chapter 6

Treatment – the patient journey

OVERVIEW

This chapter describes the typical patient journey on treatment day. It gives an insight into the working practices that are required to deliver an efficient LASIK treatment and details a typical surgical procedure so that the optometrist is well informed should the patient want to know more about the procedure itself. The patient experience during treatment is also described as it may help the patient if they are told what to expect beforehand.

CONTENTS

INTRODUCTION

Procedures do vary from clinic to clinic, and surgical techniques will differ from one surgeon to the next. The journey described is not necessarily what all clinics should do, but is an example of a typical procedure.

THE ROLE OF STAFF INVOLVED IN TREATMENT

There are usually several persons in the treatment room besides the surgeon. The patient can find this a little bewildering if it is unexpected. Below is a list of staff that are usually involved.

- **Surgeon** – An ophthalmologist carries out the surgery and oversees all aspects of the treatment.

- **Nurse** – A registered general nurse assists the surgeon and checks all equipment prior to handing it to the surgeon during treatment.

- **Overseeing nurse** – Another registered general nurse is often also present to oversee the general running of the theatre and to ensure that the needs of both the operating surgeon and assisting nurse are met.

- **Healthcare assistant** – A person is required to assist the nurse by clearing away instruments after use and to ensure that each set of equipment is sterile and set out ready for the next treatment.

- **Laser operator** – This technician ensures all the settings are correct for each patient and operates the laser computer during treatment under the direct observation of the surgeon. The laser only fires when the surgeon presses the control switch directly, thus ensuring absolute safety.

BEHIND THE SCENES PREPARATION

Clerical check

Before the treatment schedule begins, the data for patients are entered onto the laser computer by the laser operator. The treatment details are then printed off and are checked by the surgeon. The surgeon then signs the notes to acknowledge that the data entry is correct, and that no misinterpretation of handwriting has occurred.

Medication preparation

The medication for each patient to take home is prepared beforehand. Each drug must be labelled with the drug name and dose, patient's name, instructions for use and the clinic details on the actual bottles.

Surgical instrument preparation

The surgical equipment is prepared and checked. Each piece of equipment is stored until use in a sealed sterile double packet. The outer packet is removed and discarded and the remaining packet dropped onto the trolley. The inner packet is opened as and when the instrument is needed during treatment and can only be touched by a 'scrubbed' nurse or surgeon. Some of the instruments used are disposable, but items such as the microkeratome and the tonometer are sterilised and re-used in subsequent procedures. A set of equipment is used for each eye to

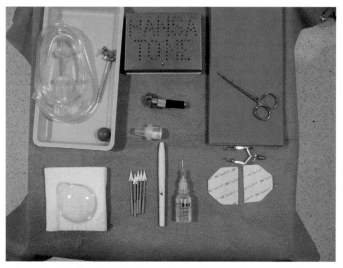

Figure 6.1   A surgical trolley that has been set up for treatment

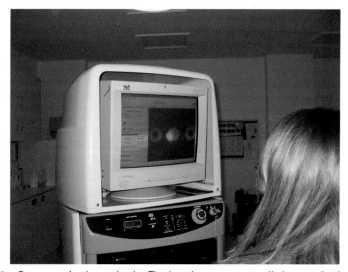

Figure 6.2   Pre-operative laser checks. The laserbeam can actually be seen in the centre of the screen

reduce the risk of cross infection between eyes. Figure 6.1 shows a typical surgical trolley that has been set up for treatment.

Laser check

The laser technician carries out a series of performance checks on the laser at the beginning of each treatment day. This involves checking the beam configuration, alignment and uniformity of transmission. Figure 6.2 shows the volume of tissue ablated per laser shot being checked. The optics and illumination systems are all checked and the tracker is also tested to ensure that it is able to lock onto the eye properly. Some settings are also checked in between each patient.

Other checks

The environmental settings of the room are also checked to ensure that the laser operates optimally. Optimum temperature and humidity requirements are specified in the laser manufacturer's instructions.

SIGNING THE CONSENT FORM

Prior to treatment day, the patient should have already read the consent form and any instructions for the day itself. The patient should be accompanied to the clinic as they will not be able to see clearly enough to drive or make their own way home easily after treatment. Some patients will also feel some discomfort for a few hours and may want some moral support from a friend or relative. The entire treatment journey takes approximately 1{½} hours.

On arrival at the clinic, the patient will be given the opportunity to raise any further questions that they may have regarding the consent form. The consent form reiterates the verbal information given at the initial consultation and should include the following:

- A statement detailing the purpose of the consent form.
- A reminder that LASIK is an elective procedure for vision correction, that other alternatives are available and that spectacles may still be required after treatment.
- An overview of the treatment procedure.
- A reminder that some discomfort or pain may occur.
- A reminder of what can be realistically expected after LASIK and that the eye changes with age.
- An explanation of the risks and complications, as well as those which are potentially sight threatening.
- Any risks specific to that patient due to other underlying factors.
- A statement which is to be signed by the patient that they have understood the information given, and they accept that as it is impossible to list every possible complication, there may further unforeseen risks that have not been stated.
- A signed statement of consent for surgery.
- A statement that is signed by the treating surgeon stating that in his opinion the patient understands the risks, benefits and potential outcomes of the procedure.

The patient may be asked to initial any points that are highlighted by the surgeon or that have been added specifically for that patient and also on each page of the consent form. This should only be done if the patient has already met the treating surgeon.

The Royal College of Ophthalmologists' guidelines indicate that the patient should attend for a consultation with the treating surgeon at least 24 hours prior to treatment if the original assessment was carried out by someone else.[1] However, this is not always the case in all clinics and, if the patient has not met the surgeon prior to treatment day, the surgeon will need to examine the patient to confirm suitability for treatment. The surgeon may wish to repeat some measurements before treatment commences (*e.g.* refraction, pachymetry). Once the surgeon has confirmed that in his or her opinion the patient has fully understood the nature of the consent form, it is then signed in the presence of that surgeon.

INSTRUCTIONS FOR AFTER-TREATMENT

A nurse or healthcare assistant will then give the patient their postoperative instructions verbally and a written copy is given to the patient to take away. Instructions include drug regimen information and general advice.

General advice and instructions for after-treatment

- Use medication as instructed on the labels.
- Use protective plastic eye shields to protect your eyes during sleep for the first night after treatment.
- Rest your eyes or go to sleep for the first few hours after treatment.
- Do not drive or work for the first day after treatment.
- Telephone the clinic or the emergency helpline if you are unsure of anything or if you are in significant discomfort.

Until medication is stopped (usually 1 week)
- Do not get any water into your eyes (avoid washing hair).
- Do not go swimming.
- Do not wear any makeup around the eyes.

For 1 month following treatment
- Do not rub your eyes.
- Do not play any contact sports.
- Avoid long-haul flights for 1 month as any dry eye will be exacerbated.

Drug regimen

The patient is instructed on how to instil eye drops safely and effectively. In most cases, the patient is given three or four types of topical drugs. Where the medication is provided in multidose bottles, the patient is given a set for each eye to reduce the risk of contamination should one eye become infected.

- **Antibiotic** (*e.g.* Exocin) – This helps to prevent microbial infection while the eye is still vulnerable. To be applied 3 times a day for 7 days unless specified otherwise by the surgeon.
- **Steroid** (*e.g.* Dexamethasone) – This is to control any postoperative inflammatory response. To be applied 3 times a day for 7 days unless specified otherwise by the surgeon.
- **Ocular lubricant** (*e.g.* Hypromellose) – This may be used 3 times day or as often as required for comfort for up to 1 month.
- **Topical Analgesic** (*e.g.* Voltorol) – In most cases this is not required and patients can take an oral medication such as Paracetamol or Ibuprofen if necessary.

All unused drugs should be returned to the clinic or a pharmacy to be destroyed. Ocular lubricants are in use for much longer, and multidose bottles can be kept for 1 month after opening.

THE TREATMENT PROCEDURE

A treatment is a common occurrence to the clinic staff, but not to the patient. Needless to say, they may be feeling nervous, excited and scared or all three emotions together and will need some re-assurance. In some cases, the healthcare assistant needs to act as a 'handholder' to give some support during the treatment. Each surgeon may have slightly different techniques that have been tried and tested with experience. The following is a typical procedure and is not specific to any particular surgeon. Further details of a typical patient experience are indicated by italics.

1. The patient is asked to lie on the treatment bed and the head is positioned so that the tracker can monitor the eye position easily. The patient's eyelid area is cleaned with an iodine solution such as aqueous povidone-iodine solution to reduce the risk of microbial contamination. One drop of topical anaesthetic is instilled in each eye. (Excessive or premature instillation may increase the risk of abrasion due to the softening effect of anaesthetic on the epithelium.)

2. The eye that is not being treated is occluded to facilitate fixation of the eye being treated which is directed at a fixation target (see Figure 6.3).

3. The surgeon isolates the eyelashes using a surgical drape or surgical tape strips and then inserts a speculum to keep the eyelids apart (see Figure 6.4). The speculum prevents the patient from blinking without causing too much discomfort and to provide a wide enough interpalprebal space to allow placement of the suction ring and use of the microkeratome.

4. The cornea and conjunctiva are irrigated with sterile salt solution to remove any conjunctival secretions. The fluid and debris may be removed using a surgical sponge spear.

5. The surgeon will use a surgical dye such as gentian violet to mark some reference points, often opposite the hinge perpendicular to where edge of the flap will be (Figure 6.5). These reference points ensure the correct repositioning of the flap especially in cases of a free cap or if cyclorotation occurs.

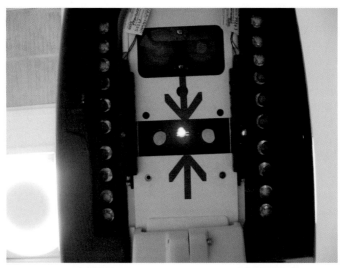

Figure 6.3   The patient is asked to fixate on the target, in this case a flashing red light

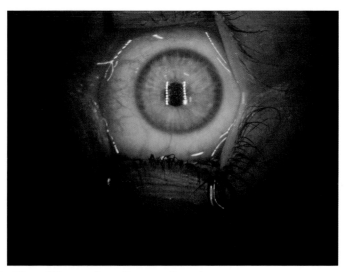

Figure 6.4   View of the eye down the operating microscope

6. The cornea is then irrigated to remove any excessive dye. Meanwhile, the microkeratome is assembled by the nurse and is checked to ensure that it is operating smoothly.

7. Further instillation of a topical anaesthetic is applied and the suction ring is then placed on the patient's eye. *If the patient has a small palprebral aperture or very tight lids, this can feel a little uncomfortable.*

8. The patient is asked to keep fixating on the fixation target. The suction is then applied and the patient is advised that their vision will temporarily fade

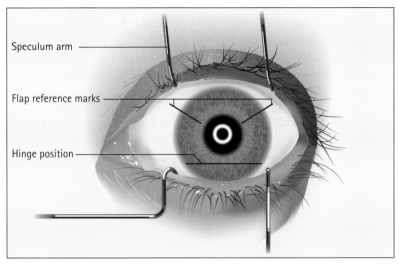

Speculum arm

Flap reference marks

Hinge position

Figure 6.5 Drawing of the eye showing the surgeon's view of the flap reference marks and hinge position

and go dark. *At this point, it is worth mentioning that the patient may find this quite frightening, and it is important to keep them calm.*

9. The surgeon checks that the intraocular pressure is sufficient (greater than 65 mmHg) using a Barraquer tonometer.

10. The eye is irrigated again with a non-saline liquid such as distilled water, and the microkeratome is placed on top of the suction ring. Sterile salt solution is not used as it may damage the microkeratome. This ensures the smooth action of the microkeratome blade and helps to prevent epithelial damage. The patient is warned that they must keep their eyes as still as possible and that they will feel a slight vibration. The microkeratome blade makes a forward and reverse pass to create a flap with a superior or nasal hinge. The suction is released and the microkeratome and the suction ring are then removed. *From a patient perspective, the most nerve wracking part of the treatment is now done and the patient can still see reasonably clearly at this point.*

11. The surgeon then uses a cannula or forceps to lift the flap and to fold it back over the hinge so that it rests on the perilimbal conjunctiva. The flap looks like a small thin soft contact lens in appearance. *The patient's vision will now feel as if they are looking through a sheet of frosted glass. However, they will still be able to see the fixation target. Due to a halo effect, the target will no longer look like a small flashing light and the patient needs to look at the centre of the target.*

12. The stromal bed is dried using an absorbent microsurgical spear and then the tracker engaged. The laser is then switched on. The surgeon maintains control of the laser function and a computer screen displays the energy emitted. A counter showing the time or percentage treatment remaining allows the surgeon to keep the patient informed as to how much longer they need to keep still. For a small prescription, the laser treatment may take less than a

minute. For high prescriptions it can be over 2 minutes. During the ablation, the surgeon ensures that the stromal bed and hinge area remain dry and that the hinge and flap are not exposed to the laser beam. *While the laser is ablating the corneal tissue, the patient cannot really tell any difference in their vision as they still have the same flashing target to look at. The patient has no sensation of the laser making contact with their eye, but they can hear a clicking sound as it is firing. The laser itself is a 'cold' laser so does not actually burn the stromal tissue, but a plume of vaporised corneal tissue is created and hence a burning odour can be smelt.*

13. Once the laser has finished, the stromal bed is evenly wetted using sterile salt solution. This allows the flap to float as it is repositioned onto the stromal bed. The flap naturally repositions itself into its original position but is gently stretched and smoothed by the surgeon to prevent striae and wrinkles. The interface is irrigated using a sterile salt solution attached to a cannula to remove any debris. The interface fluid is squeezed out and the flap smoothed down using the cannula or a spatula to ensure that it is well apposed to the stromal bed with no wrinkles. *As the flap is dried and smoothed back into position, the patient will be aware of their vision becoming clearer but still feeling watery. As the flap is being smoothed, the patient can see the instrument moving across their cornea.*

14. At the end of the treatment, the surgeon checks the flap adhesion then removes the speculum and drape. The patient is allowed to then blink, which further checks the flap adhesion. Topical medication (antibiotic and anti-inflammatory) is also applied at the end of the procedure before a plastic protective shield (Figure 6.6) is taped over the eye. *The treatment is then*

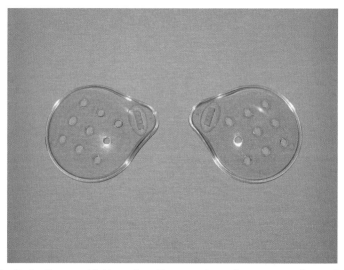

Figure 6.6 Protective eye shields such as the ones shown here are taped over the patient's eye after treatment

usually carried out on the other eye. The patient is usually less nervous by this stage, but as they know what to expect, the anticipation can make the initial parts of the procedure a little more uncomfortable.

15. When the procedure has been completed on both eyes, the patient is then accompanied back to the waiting area or to a recovery room. The patient is instructed to keep their eyes closed during the next 15–20 minutes as they may be photophobic at this stage and excessive blinking could disturb the flap.

FINAL CHECK

After approximately 20 minutes, the surgeon will examine the eyes to check that the flaps have adhered properly to the stromal bed (Figure 6.7). The vision may also be checked. The actual acuity will vary widely from person to person. In most cases it is usually around 6/36 at this stage, but in some cases the acuity can be as good as 6/7.5. Postoperative instructions are reiterated and the patient is advised to sleep for a few hours or to rest their eyes when they get home.

SHORT-TERM RECOVERY

The patient may feel varying degrees of discomfort ranging from mild grittiness to significant discomfort. The author's own experience was similar to having a dust particle underneath a rigid lens (*i.e.* extremely gritty). Once the topical anaesthetic has worn off, the degree of photophobia can be rather extreme. As a result, the patient may not be able to open their eyes at all. In such cases, the best

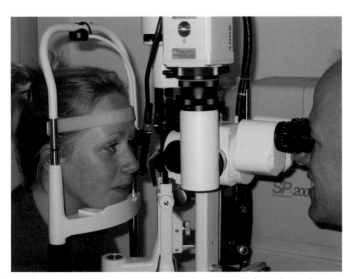

Figure 6.7   A final slit lamp examination is carried out to before the patient leaves

thing for them to do is to keep wearing dark sunglasses even indoors, and lie down with the curtains closed. If the patient is still feeling uncomfortable, then oral analgesics (such as Paracetamol or Ibuprofen) can be taken. If this is still inadequate pain relief, then 1 drop of topical Voltorol can be instilled in each eye.

After a few hours when the flap edge wound has re-epithelialized, the discomfort and photophobia will have subsided. The vision will probably have been foggy when leaving the clinic but will gradually clear as the rest of the day progresses. By the next morning, the vision should be quite good if plano was the target treatment. Many patients describe their experience of fantastic vision upon awakening, but it is worth remembering that some eyes take longer than others to recover, and it may be a few days before the vision seems clear.

In some cases, the vision after treatment is not corrected in exactly the same way as before with spectacles or contact lenses, so patients are warned to expect a few signs such as tiredness or mild frontal headaches, almost as if they are getting used to a new pair of spectacles. Haloes and glare are also common symptoms but these subside significantly after a few days. After 24–48 hours, the patient should present to the clinic for their first aftercare.

Further reading

1. Burrato S. Custom LASIK. Slack Incorporated;2003.
2. Probst LE. LASIK: a color atlas and surgical synopsis. Slack Incorporated;2003.

Reference

1. The Royal College of Ophthalmologists. Standards for laser refractive surgery. London: The Royal College of Ophthalmologists, 2003.

Chapter **7**

Postoperative assessment

OVERVIEW

This chapter covers the potential symptoms that a typical patient may experience. Each symptom is discussed so that the optometrist can reassure the patient appropriately. Typical clinical findings that an optometrist may encounter while postoperatively managing patients are also included. Complications that may require ophthalmologist intervention are covered in Chapter 8.

CONTENTS

INTRODUCTION

The optometrists' role in postoperative care can vary widely according to whether they are working in their own practice, or whether they are in a clinic. It will also vary according to whether the patient will see both optometrist and ophthalmologist on the same aftercare appointment. The first aftercare is usually carried out by the surgeon, although optometrists may carry out some part of this first aftercare. In most cases, the optometrist is the only professional that the patient sees at subsequent aftercares, but it is The Royal College of Ophthalmologists' view that the responsibility for the postoperative care of the patient remains with the ophthalmologist that carried out the treatment.[1] With this in mind, it would be sensible to presume that the optometrist should carry out whatever tests that are required by the treating ophthalmologist or clinic. As the management strategy can vary according to the optometrist's findings, each potential scenario should be clearly discussed between surgeon and optometrist before the duty of postoperative care is delegated. As discussed previously, there should be protocols in place for all shared-care schemes.

FOLLOW-UP SCHEDULE

The patient may present for their first aftercare between 1 and 3 days of treatment. The Royal College of Ophthalmologists' guidelines have previously suggested that the patient should be routinely followed up according to the following schedule:

> After 1 day
> After 7–10 days
> After 6 weeks
> After 3 months
> After 6 months
> Discharge 12 months

However, some surgeons prefer to check the eye after 48 hours instead of the next day. There are advantages to both aftercare strategies.

First, assume that aftercare is carried out according to the next-day and one-week regimen. From a patient perspective, it is re-assuring to have one's eyes checked the next day and to be told that everything is fine. Measurement of the vision the next day is also more convenient if the patient is keen to return to work as soon as possible or to drive. It is also presumable that if any striae are present, or if there are disturbances in the flap, the sooner they are rectified after treatment, the better the likely visual outcome. However, postoperative inflammation and infection does not usually present until after 48 hours and could be left to deteriorate for up to a week unless the patient presents to the clinic or their optometrist. The success of this aftercare regimen is, therefore, dependent upon the patient noticing any signs or symptoms and then presenting themselves to the clinic should problems arise. This cannot be depended upon as LASIK patients may easily confuse normal post-surgical signs and symptoms with those of complications and simply think that their eyes are 'just settling down'.

Alternatively, if a patient is seen 2 or 3 days postoperatively, most cases of infection or inflammation would still be detected at an early stage and dealt with appropriately. If the flap is accidentally displaced, it can still be easily lifted and repositioned for up to several days after treatment. If the flap displacement is quite severe and requires more urgent attention, the patient is likely to present at the clinic as the symptoms are more noticeable (*e.g.* increased discomfort, deterioration of the vision). Significant striae or wrinkles can also be easily smoothed. The earlier this is done, the better the prognosis for the patient's visual recovery. With regards to the above aftercare schedules, there is no right or wrong, and the optometrist is best guided by the treating ophthalmologist.

TYPICAL SYMPTOMS

The surgeon usually carries out the first aftercare following treatment but may delegate some part to an optometrist. As with any check-up, it is usual to start by asking about any signs and symptoms. In most cases, the patient will report that their eyes are comfortable and that their vision is good. However, there are several variations of this that can still be normal in postoperative recovery. In order to identify anything suspicious, it is necessary to know the typical signs and symptoms that a patient may experience in the early stages of recovery. These are summarised in Table 7.1.

Table 7.1 Normal postoperative symptoms

Symptom	Possible causes	Resolution
Haloes, veiling glare, starburst	Corneal oedema or small optic zone size. Corneal clarity not yet recovered	Rapid improvement initially, then a slower rate of change for up to 12 months[3]
Fluctuating vision	Corneal oedema, dry eye or residual myopia	Usually within 1–3 months
Reduced night vision	Reduction in contrast sensitivity	Returns to pre-operative levels after 6 months[4,5]
Gritty or dry eye	Keratectomy results in corneal nerve fibres being severed and corneal desensitisation	Usually between 2–12 months[6,7]
Frontal headaches or tiredness	Change in binocular balance compared with spectacles or contact lenses. Possible change in convergence demand for near tasks compared with spectacles	Like adjusting to a new pair of spectacles, it can take a couple of weeks. May require convergence exercises

Within an hour of treatment, the patient will have noticed some ocular discomfort when the topical anaesthetic has worn off. The degree of pain can be very variable and where some patients may only notice a mild irritation, others may feel significant discomfort. The patient may also have experienced in varying degrees of severity: photophobia, foreign body sensation, excessive lacrimation, hazy vision and tiredness. The patient may have needed to use topical or systemic analgesics if in discomfort, or if in pain, a topical analgesic may have been necessary.

The next day, the patient may still feel a little delicate, but ocular comfort should have returned without excessive photophobia. The vision will be much clearer although some of the following symptoms will still be noticed.

Visual disturbance

Haloes, veiling glare and starburst may be experienced in varying degrees by the patient. It is particularly noticeable in the first 48 hours and is due to post-surgical corneal oedema. Where there are several light sources close together such as with traffic signals, the halo around each source can overlap with quite dramatic effects. The symptoms recede as corneal clarity is restored and any residual effects are minimal after a few weeks although improvements are possible for up to 12 months. Where they do persist, it is often due to haze or the treatment optical zone edge falling within the scotopic pupil.[3]

Reduced night vision

Contrast sensitivity is lowered temporarily after treatment while the cornea recovers. Any decrease in corneal clarity caused by treatment, even if it is only slight can have an effect on the contrast sensitivity of the eye. Patients may, therefore, notice that their vision is better in good natural light than under artificial or poor lighting conditions. Contrast sensitivity returns to pre-operative levels after 6 months in most eyes.[4,5]

Fluctuating vision

Insufficient tear production or poor tear quality is a major cause of fluctuating vision in the early stages of recovery. Corneal oedema or disturbance can also be a factor in some patients which can induce a temporary refractive error. In most cases, the cornea settles and oedema resolves during the first 48 hours after treatment.

Gritty or dry eye

Keratectomy results in some corneal nerve fibres being severed which results in desensitisation. This disruption to the feedback loop controlling tear production can cause a foreign body sensation and may result in corneal desiccation. Where the corneal epithelium is severely affected, the patient may complain of blurred vision and sore eyes. This usually resolves within 3 months but can take longer.[6,7] The recovery period is highly variable from one individual to the next with females being generally slower to recover than males.

Frontal headaches or tiredness

Patients can sometimes suffer from asthenopic symptoms for a few days after surgery. This may be due to a change in how their vision is binocularly balanced compared to what they were accustomed to in spectacles or contact lenses. Previously myopes may also have an increased convergence demand for near tasks compared to when corrected with spectacles. In most cases, the patient adapts just as they would with a new pair of spectacles and symptoms resolve in a couple of weeks.

VISION ASSESSMENT

Patient psychology

This is quite often an emotional point for the patient as it can answer their high hopes or confirm their worst fears about the outcome of treatment. Most patients will have 6/18 acuity or better at this stage, but it is worth considering the patient's answers to how their eyes have been when taking symptom history. If they are happy and enthusiastic about their vision, then it is possible to assume that the acuity will be quite good. If they are reserved about their vision it may be that they genuinely do not know how good their vision is, or at the opposite end of the scale, that they are in denial about their vision being less than hoped for. Some patients state quite clearly that their vision is blurred. This would normally mean that the acuity is low; however, in some cases, the acuity is high and the patient has unrealistic expectations. If there is any doubt about the acuity it is best to start the patient with the larger Snellen letters. Just as with low-vision patients, there is nothing worse for the patient than to be asked to read the bottom line and not be able to.

Measuring acuity

Distance and near acuity as well as the acuity at any relevant working distance for the patient (*e.g.* VDU) should be measured. The patient should be encouraged to try and read to the best line of acuity. The result is an indicator of effectivity of the surgery, as well as giving the patient a psychological boost if they are seeing very well. Quite often a patient will be vaguely pleased with their vision when they enter the consulting room, but delighted when they leave if they have been told they can read the equivalent to 20/20. Presbyopes that have not opted for monovision should be advised to use ready readers temporarily while their vision continues to settle down.

Management of vision and residual refractive error

Although refraction can be highly variable in the early stages of recovery, it can give an indication of how the patient has responded to treatment. It gives more information than vision, as any patient with accommodation can focus through a moderate amount of hypermetropia. It is common to find some ammetropia at this stage and even some induced astigmatism. It is important not to dwell on the actual amount of correction at this stage as any prescription found may well disappear over the next few weeks. If the patient is informed of an induced astigmatism where there was none before treatment, they quite often over-react and become concerned. So it is best to be tactful and explain the results clearly, should the patient ask questions.

Hypermetropes tend to be slightly overcorrected initially (*i.e.* myopic) and find that the near vision is better than anticipated and the distance a little worse. This is more noticeable in hypermetropic patients who were previously under corrected with spectacles. For hypermetropes, the distance vision generally improves over the following month, but near vision worsens slightly if they are presbyopic, and a reading correction is required. Myopes generally tend to have a speedier visual recovery than high astigmats and hypermetropes. However, myopes that were previously accustomed to removing their spectacles for close work may find the change in accommodative demand slightly tiring. It is important to inform patients of what to expect so as to re-assure them as they experience their individual visual recovery. For those patients who complain of blurred vision even when they can see 6/6, it is best to remind them that for their first aftercare, the vision is very good indeed and that as the eyes continue to recover, the quality of vision will improve.

Where vision is not at the required level for the patient's visual tasks, it may be necessary to prescribe some temporary spectacles. It should be emphasised to the patient that as the cornea is still settling, the prescription may change and that spectacle lenses occasionally need to be replaced more than once. In most the cases, the prescription decreases over the first few weeks, especially where there is a moderate cylindrical component. Therefore, it is advisable to modify the prescription if possible to aid adaptation and to minimise replacement lens costs. The issued prescription should have the usual information, as well as indicating that it is a temporary prescription following refractive surgery.

OCULAR EXAMINATION

This should be carried out by the optometrist or the surgeon.

Lids and lashes

Patients will have been advised not to wash their eyes for the first week at least and lash deposits may be significant from the eye drops being used (Figure 7.1). It may be appropriate to instruct the patient to clean their eyelashes with cotton

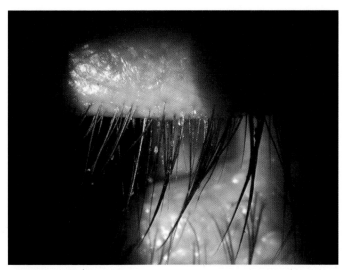

Figure 7.1   Lash deposits

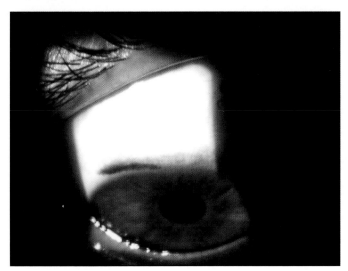

Figure 7.2   Subconjunctival haemorrhage at 1 month

buds and cooled boiled water to loosen the crusts formed. Blepharitis should not be an issue as it is normally treated prior to surgery, and postoperative treatment regimens routinely include an antibiotic.

Conjunctiva

The bulbar conjunctiva may show some subconjunctival haemorrhages which are a result of the pressure applied by the suction ring during treatment. Most patches will clear in a few days, although if the area is extensive, it may take a few weeks to clear completely (Figure 7.2). The patient should be re-assured appropriately.

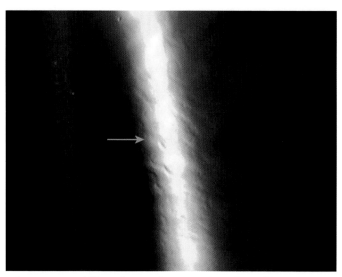

Figure 7.3   An orange peel like reflex on the cornea is typical of flap oedema

Cornea

The cornea itself can vary greatly in appearance from one patient to the next. Some corneas will look extremely clear, as if no treatment has been done at all. Some may look slightly oedematous, though not enough to cause haze (Figure 7.3). Often it is the flap that is oedematous, not the stromal bed and so haze and striae may well be present, but not always linked to stromal swelling. Haze can be caused by an inflammatory response or debris. Chart 7.1 shows the differential diagnosis of postoperative corneal haze.

Interface debris   This does not usually cause any major problems unless it is on the visual axis although it may stimulate epithelial ingrowth at a later stage.[8] If the debris lies over the visual axis, it can cause some visual disturbance ranging from increased glare to a reduction in visual acuity depending upon the density and area of debris. If the amount of debris is significant, it may be worth referring to the surgeon for flap lift and irrigation. The flap can easily be lifted and the interface irrigated before smoothing the flap back into place. Where debris appears to interrupt the adhesion of the flap edge, fluorescein can be used to investigate further. If the debris is not confined to the interface, staining that is typical of a foreign body can be seen. Where this occurs, the problematic debris needs to be removed as it can provide a path of least resistance for invading micro-organisms.

Debris can come from various sources and is usually washed away before the flap is put back into place, but the stromal bed is a quite sticky and it can be difficult to wash away all traces of debris. Prolonged washing of the stromal bed is not usually done as the stroma is absorptive and can result in oedema and striae.

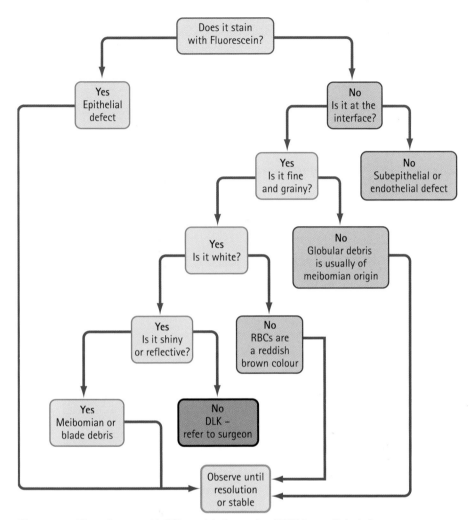

Chart 7.1 Flow chart to aid differential diagnosis of DLK from clinical signs

Sources of debris include:

- **Red blood cells** – These can be seen at the interface between the flap and the stromal bed which result from neovascular structures being severed when the flap is cut during treatment. They appear a reddish brown colour and gradually resolve over a few weeks. Figure 7.4a shows a band of red blood cells 2 days after treatment. Figure 7.4b shows a close up of an area where contact lens induced vascularisation was present prior to treatment. The majority of the cells have been washed away, but a thin layer remains. The vision is unaffected as the cells are below the pupil margin. Neovascular structures which may have been empty prior to treatment may temporarily refill due to increased healing

(a)

(b)

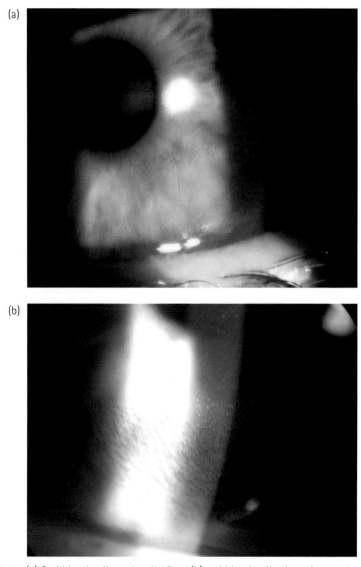

Figure 7.4 (a) Red blood cells under the flap; (b) red blood cells viewed at ×52 magnification (*continued on next page*)

activity at the flap edge. In some cases neovascularisation can also be triggered, so that new vessels follow the edge of the flap (Figure 7.4c). The vessels have usually emptied by 3–6 months postoperatively.

- **Meibomian secretions** – The appearance can vary greatly depending upon the amount of debris present. When plentiful it forms a flat, pale grey mass with indistinct edges and can appear to have small shiny globules within it

(c)

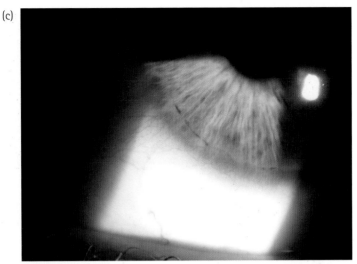

Figure 7.4 (c) Neovascularisation near the flap edge with some 'pooling' of cells in the gutter (*continued from previous page*)

(a)

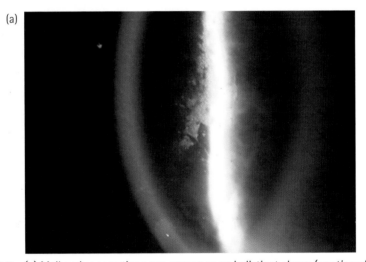

Figure 7.5 (a) Meibomian secretions can appear as an indistinct clump (*continued on next page*)

(Figure 7.5a). Other times, when most of the secretions have been washed away, the debris can look like an oily smear (Figure 7.5b). A careful section of the cornea reveals that the debris to be under the flap and not in the tear film. Again, the debris gradually resolves over time.

- **Surgical debris** – This is not unusual and can come from any of the surgical equipment used. Figure 7.6a shows at ×50 magnification where a

(b)

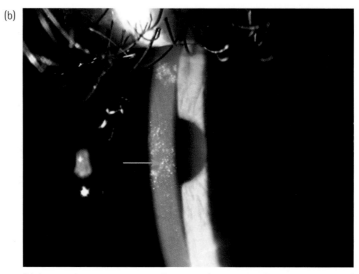

Figure 7.5 (b) It can also appear as an oily smear (*continued from previous page*)

(a)

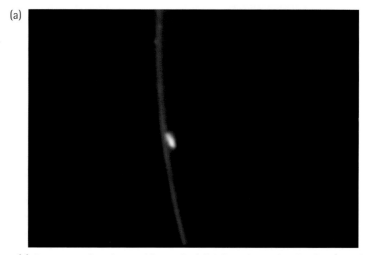

Figure 7.6 (a) A cross section shows this surgical debris to be under the flap (*continued on next page*)

fibre from a swab has stuck to the stromal bed. Such debris is inert and if it is not on the visual axis, it is better to leave it alone than to start lifting a flap that has settled well. Figure 7.6b shows debris from a similar source, but the fibre lies close to the flap edge. In this case, the surgeon decided to remove it. It is also possible to see within the interface, a scattering of very small reflective particles (Figure 7.6c). The appearance is similar to that of tear

(b)

(c)

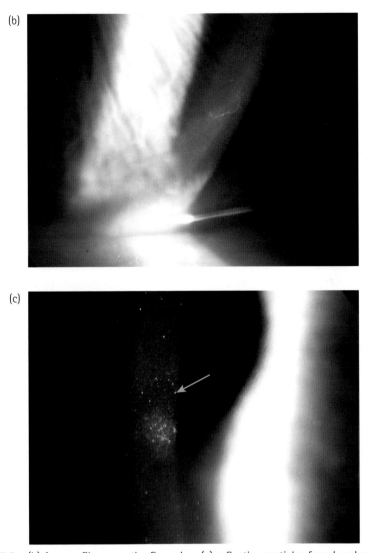

Figure 7.6 (b) A swap fibre near the flap edge; (c) reflective particles found under the flap are most likely to be from the microkeratome blade (*continued from previous page*)

film specular debris. These metallic particles are thought to be from the microkeratome blade and again do not cause any problems as they are inert.

Haze This can be caused by an inflammatory response, the onset of which is 48–72 hours after treatment with the patient becoming symptomatic in most cases. The severity of symptoms depends upon the progress of the inflammation.

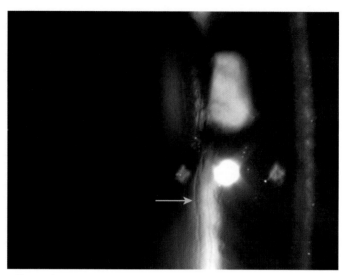

Figure 7.7 Flap striae seen at the first postoperative visit

This complication is called diffuse lamellar keratitis (DLK) and is discussed in the next chapter.

Striae These should to be evaluated carefully as the depth will differentiate between oedema of the stromal bed and flap disturbance. Striae may occur as the flap settles (see Figure 7.7) or if the flap is slightly displaced. Some striae can barely be seen as they do not look like solid structures within the stroma, but like an uneven glass pane. A wavy appearance can sometimes be seen with negative fluorescein staining as shown in Figure 7.8. It shows that the flap is not completely flat and the flap edge can also be seen even though it does not stain. Striae can occur as the flap settles, and the greater the degree of ablation, the more likely it is that micro-striae will appear in the flap. This is due to the stromal bed being ablated to a different shape and the flap no longer fits over it perfectly. If these striae do not cause a disturbance in the vision and the acuity is good, the surgeon is unlikely to take any action at this stage. Visually significant flap striae and wrinkles are discussed in the next chapter.

Desiccation This is a common side effect of LASIK and is due to corneal nerve fibres being divided when the flap is cut. Patients will have been warned to expect some dry eye symptoms and to use their artificial tears at least 3 times a day. The severity of dry eye can vary widely between patients, with some only having mild inferior staining (see Figure 7.9) and others having superficial punctuate keratopathy. If the patient has significant discomfort or if the vision is impaired, the use of gel-based eye lubrication may improve things. Management of severe dry eye is discussed in Chapter 8. In most cases, the use of artificial tears is

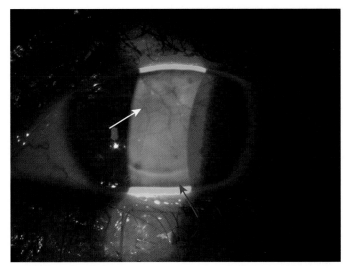

Figure 7.8 Negative fluorescein pooling shows the change in curvature at the flap edge (red arrow). Microstriae can affect the regularity of the flap and cause a consistent pattern of uneven tear film break-up (white arrow). This is common after large myopic treatments

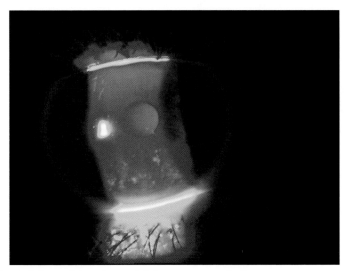

Figure 7.9 Inferior staining observed 2 days postoperatively

only required for 6–8 weeks and the patient should be re-assured that their symptoms will decrease with time.

The first aftercare should finish by reminding the patient of their post-operative instructions so as to increase the likelihood of compliance. This should include medication instructions and advice about avoiding the risk of infection or discomfort.

SUBSEQUENT AFTERCARES

One month aftercare

- **Vision** – By one month, the vision should be fairly stable and the acuity at this stage is a good indicator of the final acuity that the patient will achieve. If there is a significant refractive error, the patient should be informed that a second LASIK treatment may be necessary. The decision to re-treat is not taken until the cornea is well settled, usually after a minimum of 3 months postoperatively.

- **Conjunctiva** – Any subconjunctival haemorrhages should be reabsorbed or well on their way to being clear by one month.

- **Cornea** – Any debris of ocular origin should be almost clear by this stage. Foreign debris such as surgical fibre is sometimes surrounded by a localised area of diffuse opacification which is not usually significant. However, late onset DLK can occur so it is best to record all corneal signs. Delayed onset DLK is a rare complication[8–10] but early diagnosis and referral is essential to minimise any risk to the vision. The interface should be examined for any signs of epithelial ingrowth which usually appears at the flap edge and may be associated with episodes of DLK or debris.[11] This is caused by epithelial cells growing under the flap at the interface, usually progressing from the edge of the flap. In appearance, the ingrowth looks like oil droplets under the flap (Figure 7.10a) and can also take on a milky appearance (Figure 7.10b). The epithelial ingrowth usually stabilises without further progression. However, if it is on the visual axis or appears progressive, it may result in a thinning or melting of the overlying flap and removal is necessary. This is discussed in Chapter 8.

Final aftercare

By 3–6 months, the eye should have settled adequately to determine if discharge is appropriate. Where the post-LASIK eye is quiet at 3 months and all signs are stable, further complications are unlikely.

- **Vision** – A comparison between the best corrected acuity before and after treatment will indicate how the patient has recovered from treatment. It is particularly useful at the 3-month stage in determining if the visual recovery is satisfactory prior to deciding on re-treatment or discharge. If the patient is not satisfied with the acuity, further treatment may be possible when the cornea has stabilised. The criteria for further treatment are discussed in Chapter 9.

- **Cornea** – Epithelial ingrowth should be receding at this stage. Interface meibomian debris at this stage should be minimal and will continue to resolve. The flap edge should be smooth with no fluorescein staining or pooling. Some corneas will have healed with almost no scarring at all, whereas others will have a significant degree of fibrosis. Figure 7.11 shows an uncomplicated flap that has healed well with only minimal scarring. Dry eye signs and symptoms

(a)

(b)

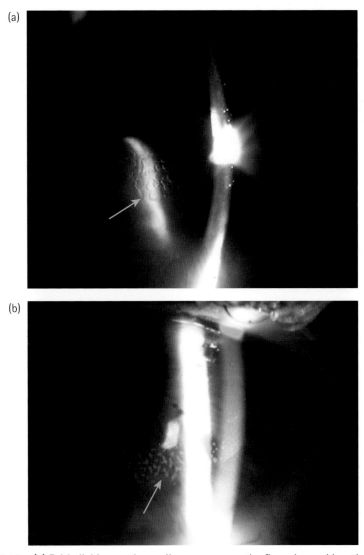

Figure 7.10 (a) Epithelial ingrowth usually appears near the flap edge and has the appearance of oil droplets on water; (b) it may have a milky appearance

are usually negligible by three months and, if the patient is still suffering, discharge should be postponed until their condition is stable.

- **Conjunctiva** – Any subconjunctival haemorrhages should now be clear and neovascular areas of the limbus that were active at 1 month will also be quietening down. Occasionally, the increased vascular response after treatment will induce neovascular growth along the flap edge (Figure 7.12). Once the cornea has healed, the vessels will empty.

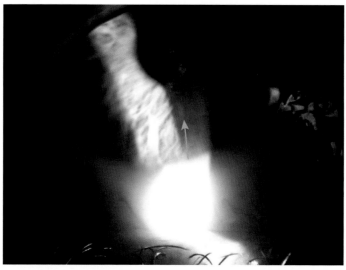

Figure 7.11 A normal flap edge 3 months postoperatively

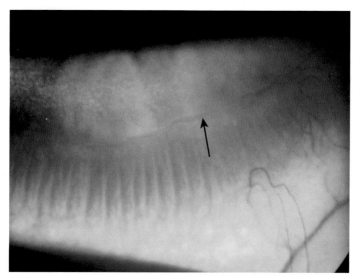

Figure 7.12 This once filled blood vessel has now emptied

On discharge, the patient usually wants to know their acuity and prescription details. It is worth pointing out to presbyopic patients that the refraction result is not necessarily a prescription for spectacles, particularly if they have precise occupational near-vision requirements. It is best to forward this information to both their GP and optometrist together with pre- and postoperative intraocular pressure details (see Chapter 9). This will ensure continuing care of the patient.

References

1. The Royal College of Ophthalmologists. Excimer laser photo-ablative surgery: best clinical practice guidelines. London: The Royal College of Ophthalmologists, 1998.
2. The College of Optometrists. Advice for fellows and members – photorefractive keratectomy. The College of Optometrists, 1995.
3. Fan-Paul NI, Li J, Miller JS *et al.* Night vision disturbances after corneal refractive surgery. Surv Ophthalmol 2002;47:533–546.
4. Montes-Mico R, Charman WN. Choice of spatial frequency for contrast sensitivity evaluation after corneal refractive surgery. J Refract Surg 2001;17:646–651.
5. Chan JW, Edwards MH, Woo GC *et al.* Contrast sensitivity after laser *in situ* keratomileusis, one-year follow-up. J Cataract Refract Surg 2002;28:1774–1779.
6. Ang RT, Dartt DA, Tsubota K. Dry eye after refractive surgery. Curr Opin Ophthalmol 2001;12:318–322.
7. Battat L, Macri A, Dursun D, Pflugfelder SC. Effects of laser *in situ* keratomileusis on tear production, clearance, and the ocular surface. Ophthalmology 2001;108:1230–1235.
8. Buxey K. Delayed onset diffuse lamellar keratitis following enhancement LASIK surgery. Clin Exp Optom 2004;87:102–106.
9. Asano-Kato N, Toda I, Tsubota K. Severe late-onset recurrent epithelial erosion with diffuse lamellar keratitis after laser *in situ* keratomileusis. J Cataract Refract Surg 2003;29:2019–2021.
10. Amano R, Ohno K, Shimizu K *et al.* Late-onset diffuse lamellar keratitis. Jpn J Ophthalmol 2003;47:463–468.
11. Asano-Kato N, Toda I, Hori-Komai Y *et al.* Epithelial ingrowth after laser *in situ* keratomileusis: clinical features and possible mechanisms. Am J Ophthalmol 2002;134:801–807.

Chapter **8**

Postoperative complications

OVERVIEW

This chapter covers the potential complications that an optometrist may encounter. Most postoperative complications occur within the first month of surgery, but late-onset occurrences of some conditions are possible. If the patient has been discharged or is being co-managed, the optometrist may be the first ophthalmic professional to detect the complication. As some of the complications are potentially sight-threatening, it is important that the optometrist is able to recognise the early signs and symptoms so that appropriate referral to the surgeon can be made.

CONTENTS

THE OPTOMETRIST'S ROLE

As optometrists may be the first ophthalmic professionals to see the patient postoperatively, it is important that they are able to recognise the clinical signs of potential complications. It is also possible that a patient may present to an optometrist's practice in an emergency if they live far away from the clinic that carried out the treatment. Correct recognition of signs and appropriate management can prevent complications from having a severely detrimental effect on the visual outcome.

In most cases, the management of complications is carried out by the surgeon, but the optometrist needs to know when it is appropriate to refer to the surgeon and what the likely management will be. Where it is not possible to refer back to the treating surgeon, it may be appropriate to refer for local ophthalmologist opinion in an emergency. Where an optometrist is co-managing a patient under normal circumstances, it is The College of Optometrists' view that the responsibility of the patient remains with the treating surgeon.[1]

The typical aftercare patient presenting to an optometrist in their own practice or in a satellite clinic where there is no surgeon present is usually uncomplicated. Urgent complications requiring immediate surgeon intervention usually manifest themselves within the first week after treatment when the patient is seen in the clinic environment. By the time the patient is attending for 1-month aftercare in a satellite practice, the eyes are usually quiet and the optometrist needs only to keep good records.

In instances where the optometrist needs to provide a topical agent, the rules regarding the sale and supply of drugs applies as in routine practice.[2] A list of drugs that an optometrist can use can be found in the *Optometrists' Formulary* issued by The College of Optometrists.[3] The topical agents that may be required in LASIK co-management are listed in Table 8.1.

Before prescribing any form of drug, it is best to confirm that the patient's medical history has not changed since it was originally checked by the treating clinic. For example, a female patient may have become pregnant since having treatment, in which case even some of the artificial tears are not recommended by the manufacturer due to the presence of preservative agents.

Table 8.1 The following topical agents are listed in the Optometrists' Formulary, and can be used to postoperative manage patients

Artificial tears	Antimicrobials
Liquid paraffin (Lacri-Lube)	Chloramphenicol
Carbomer 980 (Geltears, Viscotears)	Framycetin
Polyvinyl alcohol (Hypotears, Sno tears)	Dibromopropamidine
Hypromellose (Ispto Alkaline)	Brolene ointment
Povidone (Oculotect)	Propamidine (Brolene)
Hydroxyethylcellulose 0.44%	

MICROKERATOME-RELATED COMPLICATIONS

Optometrists working within clinics and examining patients soon after treatment may see the following complications. It is unlikely that they will be required to manage the complication as a surgeon is usually in attendance.

Failed flap

There are several possible causes of a failed flap: incomplete suction, the patient squeezing their eyes together and displacing the microkeratome, malfunction of the microkeratome, or an epithelium that has a tendency to be loose. Fortunately, such incidences are rare with one study quoting all flap complications to be 2.19%.[4]

Symptoms   When a flap failure occurs, treatment is aborted and the failed flap is left to heal. Apart from the vision, the eye will feel no different to the eye that has had successful treatment. In some cases, if abrasion has occurred, there may be some foreign body sensation.

Signs   The appearance of a failed flap can vary in appearance depending upon its nature. The flap could be too thin, too small, misplaced or mishappen (Figure 8.1). When examining the cornea, it is possible to see the irregular or misplaced outline of the flap edge (Figure 8.2).

Management   For the patient, a failed flap can be upsetting, frustrating and disappointing. In such cases it is important to emphasise that although this is a complication, the cornea will heal and treatment can still be done in the near future. The patient must realise that the final visual outcome of their treatment is unlikely to be affected. The priority here is on ensuring that the patient is comfortable and that the flap heals satisfactorily. A second treatment attempt can be made after the appropriate recovery period (usually 3 months' minimum).

Another consideration is that as most patients have bilateral treatment, the other eye will probably have had a successful outcome. If the patient is unable to suppress the non-corrected eye, it may be necessary to prescribe temporary spectacles to correct any resultant anisometropia. Some patients may prefer not to have a correction if their other eye is seeing very well as aniseikonia may be more difficult to deal with than suppressing a blurred image. When the risk of postoperative infection is over, and the cornea is reasonably settled, the surgeon may allow the eye to be fitted with a soft contact lens temporarily to resolve any symptoms.

Epithelial complications

Abrasions can occur when the microkeratome cuts the flap. There are some predisposing characteristics that increase the risk:

- **Age** – There is a linear increase in basement membrane thickening with age and, after the age of 45 years, there is an increased risk of abrasions.

(a)

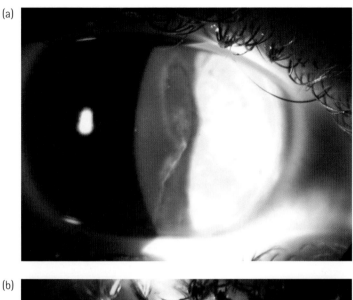

(b)

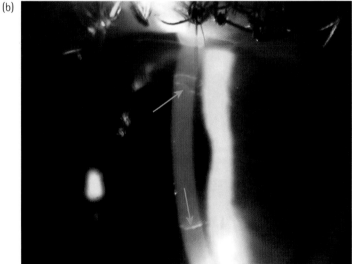

Figure 8.1 (a) Flap buttonhole as seen at first postoperative visit; (b) resolving flap complication

- **Diabetes** – A thickened basement membrane increases the risk of abrasion and a reduced rate of epithelial regeneration results in an higher risk of other post-operative complications such as infection.

- **Epithelial toxicity** – Several topical agents are used during the treatment process to which a patient's cornea may react. The resultant epithelial irregularity (Figure 8.2a) may pre-dispose the cornea to an abrasion.

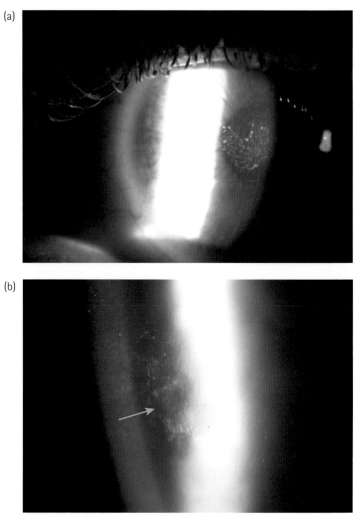

Figure 8.2 (a) Epithelial defect following an abrasion, with mild toxicity reaction; (b) epithelial abrasion after 48 hours

Symptoms The patient may have a foreign body sensation depending upon the severity of the abrasion and vision may be reduced.

Signs Initially the abrasion has the usual characteristics of epithelial damage. As the damaged epithelium recovers, it appears as a raised fluffy looking semi-transparent white mass (Figure 8.2b). The defect may not stain if the surface epithelium has recovered, but a cross section indicates the depth of the damage.

Management The surgeon will have already noted the defect on treatment day and advised the patient accordingly. Action may have included a bandage contact lens, lubrication and in cases of large abrasions topical analgesics may also be indicated. The medication can be used over the contact lens. Typically, the defect heals fairly quickly, and the bandage lens is removed within 4 days.

Lubricating the eye prior to lens removal will minimise epithelial disruption. However, an excessive amount of reflex tearing can still occur and it may be necessary to wait for this to subside before attempting refraction or examination. If the symptoms do not settle within 20 minutes, the epithelium may have been slow to heal and another bandage lens may be required. The patient should be referred back to the surgeon as replacement of the lens at daily intervals may be necessary if the epithelium is slow to heal. Daily replacement minimises the risk of a toxic reaction to the build up of preservative from the topical medications.

On examination, the vision may not be very good if the abrasion lies within the pupillary area. Refraction results are unlikely to be reliable due to the uneven epithelial surface and best corrected visual acuity may well be lower than before treatment. The patient is likely to be concerned so re-assurance is necessary. After an abrasion has occurred, the vision will take longer to settle down; at this stage, the prescription and vision are not good indicators of the treatment's success. In some cases, quite high degrees of astigmatism can be induced by raised epithelium, this disappears as the abrasion resolves. The speed of recovery varies between individuals, but typical abrasions resolve within a few days.

OTHER FLAP COMPLICATIONS

Striae or displaced flap

For 24–48 hours after treatment, the flap can still be displaced by rubbing or touching the eye. To help prevent this, patients are warned and given eye shields to wear at night to prevent them from rubbing their eyes accidentally during sleep.

Symptoms   On examination, the vision tends to fluctuate and induced astigmatism or ghosting is often present. The degree of discomfort depends upon how much disturbance there has been to the flap.

Signs   When the flap has been disturbed, multiple striae/wrinkles can often be seen (Figure 8.3a). Their orientation often indicates the direction of the disturbance; in this case, the patient had rubbed their eye from the direction of the lower lid. Striae caused by physical disturbance are much more obvious than those associated with the flap merely settling onto its newly shaped stromal bed. In some cases wrinkles rather than striae are seen (Figure 8.3b).

Management   Surgical intervention is required to lift the flap and smooth out the wrinkles or striae. The flap is lifted using a cannula and the flap refloated with sterile water. The flap is smoothed back down using the long side of a saturated surgical spear. The smoothing action may need to be repeated several times to stretch out any wrinkles that are present. The sooner this is done, the better the visual prognosis. The eye then needs to be rechecked after 48 hours to ensure that the flap has resettled smoothly. Later on when the flap has settled, it may still be possible to see lines (almost like stretch marks) where the wrinkles have been smoothed out (Figure 8.3c). In most cases, they do not interfere with the vision as there is no actual disturbance of the flap itself.

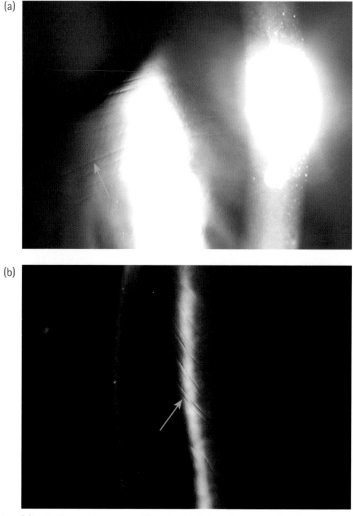

(a)

(b)

Figure 8.3 (a) Interface striae caused by physical disturbance to the flap; (b) flap wrinkles are best viewed with indirect retro-illumination (*continued on next page*)

(c)

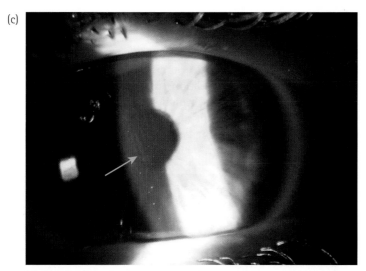

Figure 8.3   (c) The location of smoothed out striae can still be seen on this flap (*continued from previous page*)

Flap edge defect

This is not common and occurs when the flap edge is not well apposed to the stromal bed resulting in a gutter. The epithelium regrows rapidly to fill the gutter and as with other epithelial defects, there is an increased risk of epithelial ingrowth.

Symptoms   The patient is usually asymptomatic although a mild foreign body sensation may be reported.

Signs   Fluorescein floods into the gap (Figure 8.4a) and where the epithelium is penetrable, diffusion of fluorescein into the stroma will occur (see Figure 8.4b).

Management   Monitoring is required for as long as the stroma is penetrable. At this early stage of recovery, antibiotics are already being used prophylactically to reduce the risk of infection, so further medication is not required. If significant epithelial ingrowth were to occur, the flap would be relifted and the ingrowth scraped out.

EARLY POSTOPERATIVE COMPLICATIONS

Diffuse lamellar keratitis (DLK)

This is an inflammatory response that can occur after treatment which typically presents after 24 hours, although it can occur later in association with recurrent epithelial erosions.[5] It is 13–24 times more likely to occur after an epithelial defect.[6,7] (It can be confused with other corneal signs that are described in Chapter 7.

Chart 7.1 can also be used to aid the recognition of DLK to ensure appropriate management.)

Symptoms Initially, symptoms are not distinguishable from those normally experienced with dry eye. As the condition progresses, the patient becomes aware of some grittiness and photophobia, which does not ease significantly with the use of artificial tears. A worsening of the vision also occurs. In some cases, the postoperative vision can change from 6/5 to less than 6/24 in just a few days.

(a)

(b)

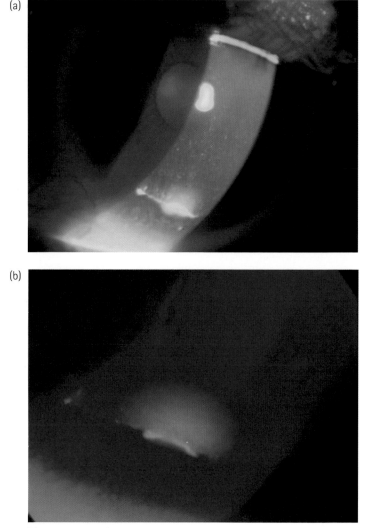

Figure 8.4 (a) Fluorescein fills the gutter between the edge of the stromal bed and the edge of the flap; (b) the edge defect allows fluorescein to penetrate into the stroma which is more noticeable after the surface fluorescein drained away

Signs   The inflammation is located at the interface between the flap and the stromal bed (Figure 8.5a) and has a dull granular appearance hence it is also known as Sands of the Sahara. Figure 8.5b shows a mild case of DLK, where a haze can be seen under the lower half of the flap. The small and fine 'grains' are close together (Figure 8.5c) and can appear almost like sand ripples in more advanced cases (Figure 8.5d). In severe cases, the DLK can make the cornea appear completely opaque.

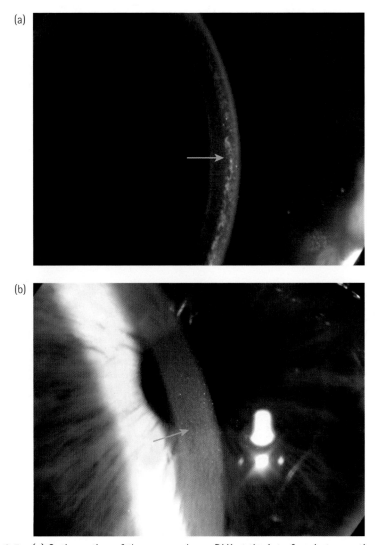

Figure 8.5   (a) Optic section of the cornea shows DLK at the interface between the flap and the stromal bed; (b) mild DLK at 48 hours – the patient was asymptomatic
(*continued on next page*)

(c)

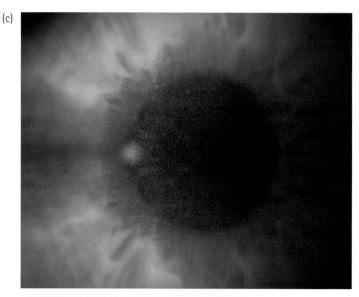

(d)

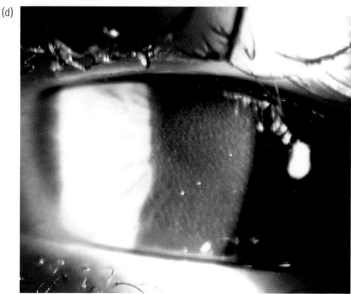

Figure 8.5 (c) Grade 1 DLK with infiltration; (d) grade 1 DLK inflammatory cells create wave-like patterns (*continued from previous page*)

Management Where DLK is suspected, referral to the surgeon is imperative as aggressive anti-inflammatory therapy may be required. This involves the use of topical steroids, the dose and frequency of which varies according to the severity of the condition. The surgeon usually examines the eye again after 48 hours to ensure that the condition is responding as expected. The medication is then tapered off over 2 weeks. In severe cases, lifting the flap and physically removing the inflammatory cells may be required.

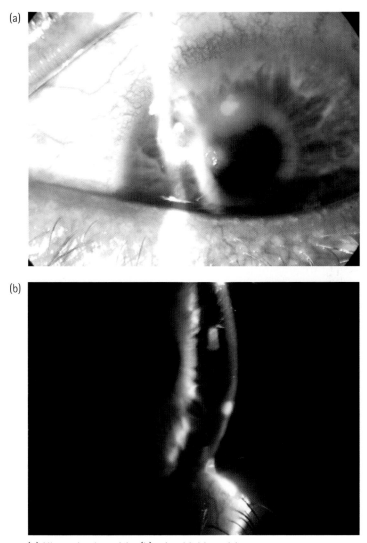

Figure 8.6   (a) Ulcerative keratitis; (b) microbial keratitis

Microbial keratitis

Antibiotics are routinely used prophylactically for one week as the eye is more susceptible to micro-organism invasion after treatment. In most cases this is adequate; however, patients are not always both compliant and hygienic, so exposure to unexpected pathogens is a possibility.

Symptoms   In LASIK patients, there is a longer period of corneal sensory denervation than in PRK[8] and some patients may not be experiencing pain or photophobia as expected. Acute onset symptoms usually present within 72 hours of surgery, but this is not always the case. Figure 8.6a shows the eye of a patient who had no sign of infection 4 weeks postoperatively, but at 8 weeks presented to the clinic complaining of only mild discomfort. The causative pathogen was not identified but it was probably a slow growing organism (*e.g. Mycobacterium* spp.)

Signs Figure 8.6b shows an early case of microbial keratitis. The corneal lesion has not yet broken the surface of the epithelium as shown by the absence of fluorescein staining. If left untreated, it could develop into an ulcer.

Management Diagnosis and treatment of postoperative infection is not within the optometrist's role and so referral to the surgeon is necessary. Treatment usually involves aggressive antimicrobial therapy. It is also appropriate to send a swab of the infected area for analysis. Where there is no surgeon on site, referral to an emergency centre would be appropriate in urgent cases. In non-urgent cases where clinical signs are minor and the patient is asymptomatic, it is advisable to speak to the treating surgeon if possible as it may be appropriate to supply or write a signed order for an antimicrobial agent. This would be for prophylactic use, to prevent the infection from worsening until the surgeon can examine the patient.

OTHER POSTOPERATIVE COMPLICATIONS

Dry eye

Disruption to the corneal nerves by the cutting of the LASIK flap results in a disturbance in the sensory feedback controlling tear production.

Symptoms Dry eye associated with pain is the most common early postoperative complication with one study reporting it in 42 out of 683 eyes that had undergone PRK or LASIK.[7] Symptoms may also worsen when the patient resumes an activity that was temporarily stopped during postoperative recovery (*e.g.* VDU use or outdoor sports, where tear evaporation increases).

Signs Practitioners are all too familiar with the typical signs associated with dry eye, but in some cases the desiccation can be severe enough to cause diffusion of fluorescein into the stroma (Figure 8.7a). It can also cause corneal oedema and induce myopia. There is no typical dry eye fluorescein pattern in eyes that have undergone LASIK. In severe cases, the entire corneal surface is covered in punctuate stain. In some cases, LASIK merely exaggerates a pre-disposition to dry eye and the staining indicates punctate epithelial keratopathy (Figure 8.7b). The staining can also appear as a central band reaching from 3 to 9 o'clock (Figure 8.7c).

Management Topical lubricants are prescribed according to the severity of patient symptoms. Hypromellose or equivalent is usually the first agent to be tried for mild-to-moderate signs of dry eye and can be used as often as required.

If the patient is not gaining adequate relief, this will be apparent by the copious amounts of lubricant they get through in the first 48 hours. For moderate-to-severe dry eye, a carbomer lubricant may improve comfort. In severe cases, a liquid paraffin-based preparation may be prescribed. Often, a battery of different lubricants is required for use at different times of the day.

In some cases, dry eye can be aggravated by preservatives in multidose containers. If the patient complains of increased discomfort or stinging immediately after insertion, it would be advisable provide a preservative free agent instead.

(a)

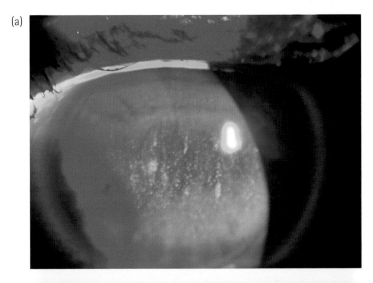

(b)

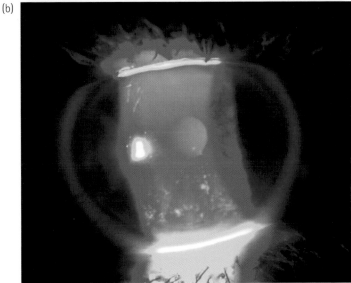

Figure 8.7   (a) Fluorescein can penetrate into the stroma with severe epithelial keratopathy; (b) inferior superficial keratopathy (*continued on next page*)

(c)

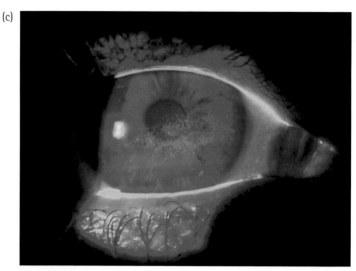

Figure 8.7 (c) Band of punctate fluorescein between 3 and 9 o'clock (*continued from previous page*)

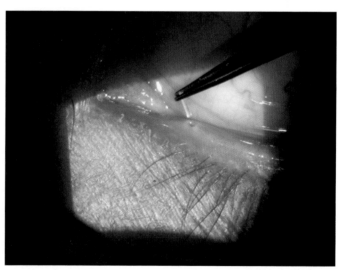

Figure 8.8 Collagen punctum plugs are inserted to give temporary relief from dry eye symptoms

Where lubricants are insufficient, temporary collagen punctum plugs can be inserted (see Figure 8.8) by either the surgeon or the optometrist (provided training has been carried out). If the symptoms are significantly reduced with the collagen plugs, silicone ones can be inserted for a semi-permanent effect. By 1 month, the dry eye symptoms ought to be reduced. By 3–6 months, symptoms are usually minimal and punctum plugs can be removed if they have not fallen out already.

Epithelial ingrowth

Signs of epithelial ingrowth may be seen at the 1 month aftercare. The incidence of epithelial ingrowth is approximately 2% but does vary according to surgical technique, microkeratome and epithelial characteristics.[9] The ingrowth tends to occur along the flap edge and is continuous with surface epithelial cells in the majority of cases.[10] It is secondary to postoperative invasion by surface epithelial cells under the flap,[5] although it is also possible by implantation during treatment. The risk of ingrowth is minimised by tight apposition of the flap to the stromal bed.

Figure 8.9a shows a significant area of epithelial ingrowth, but action is not necessary as it extends only 2 mm from the flap edge. Ingrowth is naturally self limiting and the majority of cases do not need action.[6] Epithelial ingrowth can also appear away from the flap edge at sites where debris has been present or where epithelial cells have been introduced under the flap during treatment. Epithelial cells can also migrate from the flap edge as in Figure 8.9b which shows a more aggressive ingrowth superiorly near the flap hinge. The vision was unaffected and the patient was asymptomatic. The case was referred to the surgeon for assessment. The ingrowth was non-progressive and monitoring was the only further action required.

In some cases, the cells may become necrotic and release lytic enzymes which cause flap melt. In the example shown in Figure 8.9c, the flap edge has melted leaving a widened gutter between the flap and the untreated cornea. If signs of this are seen, it must be referred to the surgeon. Where the condition is progressive, the management is to lift the flap, scrape the ingrowth out and then irrigate before replacing the flap. The patient is subsequently monitored for possible recurrence of ingrowth. Eventually, epithelial cells will fill the gutter and the epithelium will be a smooth surface.

(a)

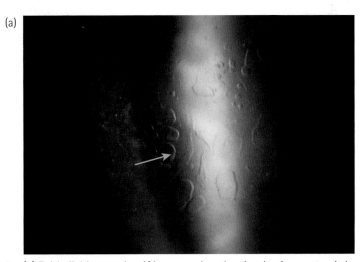

Figure 8.9 (a) Epithelial ingrowth – if it encroaches the visual axis or extends beyond 2 mm from the flap edge it may need to be removed (*continued on next page*)

(b)

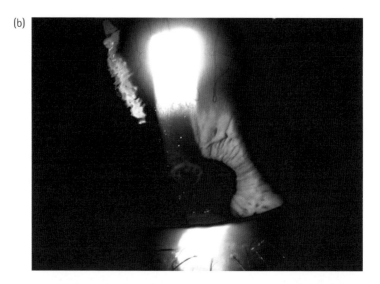

(c)

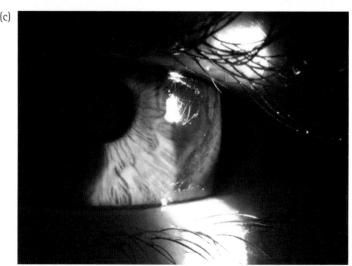

Figure 8.9   (b) Epithelial ingrowth located near the flap hinge; (c) progressive epithelial ingrowth can cause the overlying flap to melt (*continued from previous page*)

VISUAL COMPLICATIONS

High expectations that are not met

Spectacle wearers are often accustomed to a high level of corrected vision that is regularly checked and improved if necessary. Laser eye surgery aims to improve the unaided vision of the patient but it cannot guarantee to match the best corrected acuity achieved with spectacles.

Presentation The patient complains of blurred vision. A typical answer when asked about their vision is: 'I can see really well, but it's not quite right'. The unaided acuity is good, usually 6/6. There is often a small refractive error which improves the acuity to the same level as measured pre-operatively.

Management A patient may be dissatisfied if their vision is 6/6 but are accustomed to seeing 6/5 or even 6/4. This disappointment can be avoided by good pre-operative counselling about the risks associated with LASIK and ensuring that the patient understands the limitations of the treatment. Prevention is the best cure as treating small prescriptions to satisfy fussy patients is not usually worth the risk. Where it is too late for prevention, the best way to deal with a patient that is dissatisfied is to take the time to understand why they are not happy with the result.

> *Case history*
> A patient attended for a consultation with a view to having more laser eye treatment having already had LASIK elsewhere. He had complained at his last visit to the treating clinic that he was not happy with his vision. They informed him that his vision was 6/6 and that he should be satisfied. Further questioning revealed that his distance vision was not too bad but his eyes were constantly tired and he felt that he was straining to see. VDU work and reading reports were his main visual tasks. On examination, the patient was found to have vision of $6/6^{-2}$ in the right eye and 6/7.5 in the left. Refraction revealed -0.50 DC in the left eye which did not significantly change the acuity. There was also a reading addition of $+1.25$. All that was required in this case was an explanation of the visual status and advice on how to resolve the symptoms. The patient left the clinic very satisfied even though spectacles had been suggested and not more laser treatment.

In some cases, the patient merely needs to learn to live with 6/6 vision instead of 6/4. However, assumptions should not be made and ocular motor balance should be assessed in the habitual positions of gaze to ensure that decompensation of a heterophoria has not occurred by the removal of spectacles.

Unaided distance vision is lower than predicted

In the absence of other clinical signs, this may be attributed to over or under-correction by the laser treatment. It is also possible that although the resultant refractive error is zero, the patient has lost one line or more of best-corrected acuity due to induced higher order aberrations. This possibility can be investigated using wavefront aberrometry.

Presentation Patients usually give vague descriptions of being able to see, yet report the vision being blurred at the same time. If the dominant eye is affected then the reduction in vision is felt all the more keenly. In most cases, the vision is merely blurred but, occasionally, when one eye has been occluded ghosting is seen. Most patients describe ghosting as a shadow effect or a faint outline around the letters that they are reading. On examination, the vision is significantly lower than the best corrected visual acuity before treatment. A refractive error is usually found in these cases and correcting an astigmatic component often removes the ghosting. Where the acuity does not improve to a satisfactory level, the resultant blur may be due to other aberrations.

Management   At an early stage, it is best to inform the patient that the vision may take 3 months to stabilise and that the vision may well improve further during that period. Any significant refractive error that improves visual acuity can be corrected with temporary spectacles until the cornea stabilises. It is common for up to 1.00 of error to resolve by the 3-month stage; if necessary, any over or under-correction of significance can be rectified in most cases by further laser ablation (see Chapter 9). If the loss in acuity or ghosting can not be corrected with refraction, then further investigation may be required (*e.g.* wavefront aberrometry).

Unaided near vision is lower than expected

Some myopic presbyopes underestimate how the loss of their unaided near vision will feel after treatment for full correction. Other patients may have been over-corrected by the laser treatment.

Presentation   The patient does not have adequate near vision to carry out the range of near visual tasks that they require.

Management   If the patient has poor near acuity after treatment, it can come as quite a shock if they are accustomed to myopic near vision. Again, good counselling prior to treatment should help to minimise this. The patient needs to understand that the gain in the distance vision outweighs the loss of the myopic near vision. In situations where the patient cannot be reconciled to their loss of near vision, re-treatment to provide monovision may be an option.

Where the patient has been overcorrected, there is no quick fix as the treatment cannot be reversed immediately. The patient needs to be given appropriate advice with regards to near vision spectacles and in some cases varifocals can be of help. Further treatment to remove induced hypermetropia is a possibility for most patients after the cornea has stabilised.

Glare and haloes

Temporary haloes, glare and starburst are common while the cornea is settling down after treatment. Permanent visual disturbance of this nature is rare in refractive surgery where the treating ophthalmologist selects a treatment zone that provides an optical zone which is greater than the scotopic pupil. This ensures that any light scattered at the edge of the treatment zone does not enter through the pupil. Where this is not possible, the patient will have been carefully counselled prior to treatment.

An example of when this may arise is when the patient has a large scotopic pupil (*e.g.* 7.7 mm) and has a large myopic correction. If the treatment zone is set at 7.8 mm, the required ablation depth to correct the myopia may be greater than the amount of corneal tissue available to ablate. However, by reducing the treatment zone by 0.2 mm, it is possible to reduce the amount of corneal tissue required by as much as 10 μm with a −7.00 DS correction. Glare may also be induced by a hazy or scarred cornea after LASIK, although it is less common than after PRK.

Presentation   All patients are warned that they may experience haloes and glare after treatment. Some patients can have a very marked starburst or halo effect around lights whereas others have very little. In most cases, the glare is only significant for a short period of time while the cornea is settling down. In some cases there may be some disturbance to the central cornea, such as haze or debris.

Management   Patients should be informed that these visual side-effects reduce markedly in the first month and continue to resolve over a 3-month period. In some cases, the symptoms can be due to significant corneal haze or surgical debris. In such cases, lifting the flap to remove debris or controlling the haze with topical agents may be required.

Where significant haloes and glare persist, it is important to discover the extent of the symptoms and how it affects their vision – is it discomfort or disability glare? The former almost always improves by 6 months' postoperatively and re-assurance is all that is required; in the meantime, sunglasses may be effective in decreasing discomfort. For patients that complain of mild discomfort when driving under a bright but grey sky, normal sunglasses can be too dark and may impair the vision, so it would be best to suggest a tint with a greater light transmission factor.

Disability glare is difficult to solve. In many cases, quantifying the problem is difficult, as there is no current method of measuring glare in clinical practice. Glare due to the treatment zone edge being within the scotopic pupil can be reduced by fitting contact lenses which partially block out light, thus reducing the pupil diameter through which light enters.

LATE ONSET COMPLICATIONS

Late onset complications are rare but can be potentially sight threatening if not recognised and referred for appropriate management. The following complications have been reported in ophthalmic literature.

DLK

This inflammatory condition usually presents within the first few days after treatment, but can occur later in association with recurrent epithelial erosions[5,11] or after traumatic flap dislocation.[12] Referral back to the surgeon is imperative. It is managed in the same way as normal onset DLK and usually responds well to topical steroid therapy. However, some cases of late onset DLK have been associated with raised intraocular pressure that did not respond to traditional therapy and was only controlled after the intraocular pressure was lowered.[13]

Flap displacement

Experimental research has shown that although the LASIK flap can withstand 9 times the force of gravity,[14] it can still be displaced by trauma. In the cases that have been reported, the trauma has been severe and blunt (*e.g.* airbag injury[15]) or tangential, where the flap has been coincidentally shifted by force applied to a small area (*e.g.* tree branch or finger[12,16]). Visual recovery is usually successful following flap repositioning.[17,18] Immediate referral for surgeon attention is necessary for a good visual outcome. Due to minimal wound healing except at the edges of the flap, flap displacement may occur months or years after uneventful LASIK.

Iatrogenic keratectasia

This is a rare complication of ectasia is associated with a stromal bed thickness of less than 250 μm and corneal thinning dystrophies.[19] It is caused by the lowering of the strength and tension in the corneal lamellae which results in a significant increase in the curvature of the posterior and anterior corneal surfaces. It is generally accepted that the risk of ectasia is minimised by ensuring that the stromal bed remaining after ablation is at least 250 μm deep. However, current literature is unable to determine a specific residual corneal thickness or a range of pre-operative corneal thickness that would put an eye at risk. Patients usually present with blurring of the vision and topographical analysis shows progressive steepening of the cornea. Corneal suturing and intrastromal corneal rings[20–22] have been used successfully to improve the vision in these cases.

References

1. The College of Optometrists. Advice for Fellows and Members – Photorefractive keratectomy. London: The College of Optometrists, 1995.
2. The General Optical Council (Rules Relating to Injury or Disease of the Eye) Order of Council 1999, Statutory Instrument 3267.
3. The College of Optometrists. The Optometrist's Formulary. No 3. London: The College of Optometrists, 1999.
4. Lui MM, Silas MA, Fugishima H. Complications of photorefractive keratectomy and laser *in situ* keratomileusis. J Cataract Refract Surg 2003;19(2 Suppl):S247–S249.
5. Knorz MC. Flap and interface complications in LASIK. Curr Opin Ophthalmol 2002; 13:242–245.
6. Johnson JD, Harissi-Dagher M, Pineda R *et al.* Diffuse lamellar keratitis: incidence, associations, outcomes, and a new classification system. J Cataract Refract Surg 2001;27:1560–1566.
7. Shah MN, Misra M, Wihelmus KR *et al.* Diffuse lamellar keratitis associated with epithelial defects after laser *in situ* keratomileusis. Cataract Refract Surg 2000;26:1312–1318.
8. Alio JL, Perez-Santonja JJ, Tervo T *et al.* Postoperative inflammation, microbial complications and wound healing following laser *in situ* keratomileusis. J Refract Surg 2000;16:523–538.

9. Asano-Kato N, Toda I, Hori-Komai Y *et al*. Epithelial ingrowth after laser *in situ* keratomileusis: clinical features and possible mechanisms. Am J Ophthalmol 2002;134:801–807.
10. Wang MY, Maloney RK. Epithelial ingrowth after laser *in situ* keratomileusis. Am J Ophthalmol 2000;129:746–751.
11. Asano-Kato N, Toda I, Tsubota K. Severe late-onset recurrent epithelial erosion with diffuse lamellar keratitis after laser *in situ* keratomileusis. J Cataract Refract Surg 2003;29:2019–2021.
12. Aldave AJ, Hollander DA, Abbott RL. Late-onset traumatic flap dislocation and diffuse lamellar inflammation after laser *in situ* keratomileusis. Cornea 2002;21:604–607.
13. Nordlund ML, Grimm S, Lane S, Holland EJ. Pressure-induced interface keratitis: a late complication following LASIK. Cornea 2004;23:225–234.
14. Goodman RL, Johnson DA, Dillon H *et al*. Laser *in situ* keratomileusis flap stability during simulated aircraft ejection in a rabbit model. Cornea 2003;22:142–145.
15. Lemley HL, Chodosh J, Wolf TC *et al*. Partial dislocation of laser *in situ* keratomileusis flap by air bag injury. J Refract Surg 2000;16:373–374.
16. Geggel HS, Coday MP. Late-onset traumatic laser *in situ* keratomileusis (LASIK) flap dehiscence. Am J Ophthalmol 2001;131:505–506.
17. Tumbocon JA, Paul R, Slomovic A *et al*. Late traumatic displacement of laser *in situ* keratomileusis flaps. Cornea 2003;22:66–69.
18. Heickell AG, Vesaluoma MH, Tervo TM *et al*. Late traumatic dislocation of laser *in situ* keratomileusis flaps. J Cataract Refract Surg 2004;30:253–256.
19. Schmitt-Bernard CF, Lesage C, Arnaud B. Keratectasia induced by laser *in situ* keratomileusis in keratoconus. J Refract Surg 2000;16:368–370.
20. Seo KY, Lee JH, Kim MJ *et al*. Effect of suturing on iatrogenic keratectasia after laser *in situ* keratomileusis. J Refract Surg 2004;20:40–45.
21. Lovisolo CF, Fleming JF. Intracorneal ring segments for iatrogenic keratectasia after laser *in situ* keratomileusis or photorefractive keratectomy. J Refract Surg 2002;18:535–541.
22. Alio J, Salem T, Artola A *et al*. Intracorneal rings to correct corneal ectasia after laser *in situ* keratomileusis. J Cataract Refract Surg 2002;28:1568–1574.

Chapter 9

Postoperative care

OVERVIEW

Opinion varies as to when a patient should be discharged. Therefore, the postoperative care schedule should be dictated by the treating ophthalmologist. This chapter discusses the criteria that must be considered prior to discharge or further treatment. Once discharged, it is in the patient's best interests to have regular eye examinations. It is expected that relevant preoperative and postoperative data be made available to any ophthalmic professional who undertakes care of the patient in the future.

CONTENTS

INTRODUCTION

The patient is usually followed up for between 3 and 12 months after treatment. In most cases, the cornea and the vision is stable after 3 months. It is then appropriate to decide whether the patient can be discharged or whether further monitoring is required.

DISCHARGE CRITERIA

The patient is only discharged when the practitioner feels that the ocular status is stable and the patient is happy to be discharged. The following is a guide to what is expected before discharge can take place.

Vision

There is no deterioration in the unaided vision between two consecutive aftercares that are at least 1 month apart. The refractive error is considered to be stable when there is no more than 0.25 D of change in any meridian during this time.

Medication

All medication relating to treatment has been stopped. Some patients may still wish to use ocular lubricants and they should be advised on what is suitable and where it can be obtained from after discharge.

Cornea

All corneal signs should be stable.

- **Desiccation** – Tear secretions can take up to 9 months to return to pre-operative levels.[1] At discharge there should be no signs of corneal desiccation unless a history of dry eye was noted prior to surgery. If present, any corneal desiccation or dry eye symptoms should be similar to pre-operative levels. In such cases, the patient may wish to continue using artificial tears. It is appropriate to send a report to the patient's general medical practitioner documenting this information.

- **Epithelial ingrowth** – If near the edge of the flap it usually resolves or remains unchanged.[2] Where the ingrowth is more central and not continuous with the surface epithelium, it may not resolve spontaneously. There should be no signs of active epithelial ingrowth at the time of discharge. If in doubt, record the location and size of the ingrowth and review in 1 month to check for any changes.

- **Debris** – All interface debris of ocular origin fades with time and there should be no more than a minimal amount at the time of discharge. When the debris is foreign to the eye, it does not resolve and remains inert under the flap. Provided it does not interfere with the vision and there is no sign of activity localised around the debris, the patient can be discharged.

- **Haze or scarring** – Central haze is not common after LASIK; if present, the patient should only be discharged when it does not progress without being suppressed by steroidal anti-inflammatory medication. In some patients, there can be some fibrosis which is limited to a narrow band peripheral to the flap edge.[3] The scar tissue is in the corneal periphery and does not interfere with the vision.

- **Limbal vascularisation** – Any ghost vessels resulting from over wear of contact lenses that refilled after treatment should have returned to pre-treatment status.

If any of the above criteria are not met, then discharge is delayed until all signs are stable. It may also be the case that the vision is stable, but the acuity is not at a satisfactory level for the patient. In which case, further treatment may be necessary.

CONSIDERATIONS FOR RETREATMENT – OPTOMETRIST

The final decision regarding further treatment is made by the surgeon, so referral back to the treating clinic for re-assessment may be required if the optometrist is working in a satellite practice. The optometrist will need to consider the following points before referring the patient back to the surgeon for retreatment.

General health

The patient's medical history should be checked for any changes since the original treatment. If there are any circumstances that would render the cornea or refraction unstable (*e.g.* onset of diabetes or pregnancy), then referral for retreatment needs to be delayed for the appropriate period.

Motivation for retreatment

The optometrist will need to find out from the patient why retreatment is wanted and what expectations they have. If the patient has a good level of acuity but demands perfection, further treatment may not provide satisfaction. The majority of patients that want retreatment find that they are currently restricted whilst carrying out certain tasks by their vision (*e.g.* driving). For some patients, their vision may be adequate as measured by a Snellen chart, but the quality of vision may be impaired by an astigmatic or accommodative component.

Refraction

Repeat refractions at least 1 month apart should be carried out to ensure that the vision and refractive error is stable before referring on for further treatment. Where there is less than 0.75 D of refractive error, the patient may not gain much benefit from further laser ablation. However, each case is individual and refractive error is not the only deciding factor.

Visual acuity

The unaided acuity should be recorded and compared to the best corrected acuity. If there is a significant difference between them, then the patient will probably benefit from further treatment. However, if the best corrected postoperative acuity is lower than the pre-operative, then the corneal recovery may not be complete and further changes in the vision and refraction may occur. Therefore, it is best to wait until the postoperative best corrected acuity is similar to that of before treatment. In cases where there are visible causes of reduced vision (*e.g.* striae), managing those may be enough to remove the refractive error.

Presbyopia

If the patient is presbyopic or nearing presbyopia then residual/induced myopia in one or both eyes will improve the unaided near vision. The patient must understand that if the myopia is corrected, then the ability to read without spectacles will decrease. For some patients, it would be beneficial to leave one eye myopic to provide a monovision correction. If the residual error is a hypermetropic, a young patient that is able to accommodate is much more likely to tolerate it than a presbyope. Presbyopic patients who were previously myopic are extremely intolerant to overcorrection even as small as +0.50 D.

Ocular dominance

Where the dominant eye has a lower acuity than the non-dominant eye, the patient may have problems adjusting to the vision postoperatively. The patient may describe blurred vision even if they are 6/5 binocularly. The difference between the eyes may be quite small, but the patient could find it difficult to cope if there is a strong ocular dominance. If it is the non-dominant eye that is slightly myopic, it may be worth leaving the eye as it is as the patient will find it beneficial when they become presbyopic. (See Chapter 4 for more information on ocular dominance testing.)

Binocular vision status

In routine practice, optometrists ensure that the patient is binocularly balanced with their refractive correction to reduce the risk of aesthenopic symptoms. With laser eye surgery, the aim is to give the patient equivalent vision to that of their spectacles or contact lenses, but the result is not always an exact match. Most patients are happy with their vision even when one eye does not see as well as the other. However, a non-dominant eye that is not fully corrected could still cause problems if the binocular balance is upset, as a normally well-compensated heterophoria could break down. Diplopia can also become manifest after treatment if there is inadequate control of accommodation.[4]

Induced aberrations

Some patients present with stable consecutive refraction results but the best corrected acuity although stable, remains stubbornly below that of before treatment. This may be due to induced aberrations and so referral back to the treating surgeon is required to investigate the cause.

Ocular examination

If the patient's vision appears to have changed for the worse since treatment, it is important to check the ocular status to ensure that the change in vision is due to regression rather than progression of another pathology (*e.g.* cataract, macula changes). If other pathology is present, this should be dealt with in the usual way and, when resolved, the vision and refraction should be re-assessed.

CONSIDERATIONS FOR RETREATMENT – SURGEON

Once the patient has been referred back to the treating clinic, the surgeon will need to examine the patient's treatment history as well as examining the patient's eyes. Where the cause of reduced acuity is due to over or undercorrection, then the following needs to be considered.

Acuity and refractive error

The surgeon will only consider further treatment where the patient is likely to achieve a significantly improved best corrected acuity. If the unaided vision is 6/6 or better in the eye to be retreated, then the risks associated with surgery, although they are small, could outweigh the potential benefits.

Corneal thickness

Ultrasound pachymetry will have been carried out prior to surgery and the depth of tissue ablated will have been recorded. It is, therefore, possible to calculate the residual cornea and to deduce whether further treatment is possible. However, the surgeon will measure the corneal thickness again to ensure that the information used to in the retreatment calculation is accurate.

Example calculation
Pre-operative corneal thickness = 510 μm
First treatment ablation = 60 μm
Microkeratome setting for flap thickness = 180 μm
Residual stromal thickness = 510 − 60 − 180 = 270 μm
Ablation depth required for further treatment = 9 μm
Final residual stromal thickness = 270 − 9 = 261 μm

In some cases, where the original prescription was high or if the cornea was thinner than average, there may not be enough corneal tissue left to provide a further treatment safely. The criterion for the residual stromal bed is the same as for original treatment; that is it must be at least 250 μm thick to minimise the risk of ectasia. The calculations assume that each LASIK flap is cut a determined thickness by the microkeratome (*e.g.* 180 μm). However, studies have shown great variability in flap thickness even when the microkeratome has been set to cut flaps of the same thickness.[5]

In many cases the flap is thinner, so the stromal bed is likely to be thicker than calculated. It is also possible that the flap may be thicker[6] and where this occurs, the residual stromal bed may be thinner than expected. The only way of knowing if further treatment is possible is to lift the flap and measure the stromal bed underneath. Accurate assessment of residual stromal thickness is essential to avoid the risk of ectasia and possibly perforation in extreme cases.[7] If the measurement is equal or greater than the ablation depth required plus 250 μm for the residual bed, then treatment can proceed.

Topography and wavefront aberrometry

The cornea also needs to be stable and the surgeon should check topographic images of the cornea to identify any irregularities before further treatment. This is important as the patient's blurred vision may not be purely due to refractive error. Irregularities such as central islands or peninsulas can occur which can be seen on topographical maps as localised areas of steepening on a flattened central cornea. These arise due to underablation in a localised area of the stromal bed. Studies indicate the cause to be related to the use of broad-beam lasers and the plume that is given off during treatment.[8] Advances in laser technology have resulted in this complication being much less common.

Corneal topography would also show if there are any areas where the cornea is more raised, or if the ablation is decentred. The latter is rarely found now due to the use of sophisticated eye-movement trackers installed with laser systems. However, subtle irregularities which cause higher order aberrations may not be detected by topography. Where visual signs cannot be solved by two spectacle prescription, investigation with wavefront aberrometry is required. Any significant higher order aberrations found will need to be taken into consideration along with the prescription details.

COUNSELLING

If the patient is deemed to be suitable for further laser treatment, the surgeon will then discuss the procedure and any associated risks and benefits.

Risks and benefits

The surgeon will discuss these with the patient, and where the residual error is quite small the patient needs to be aware that an improvement is not guaranteed. There are three possible outcomes:

- The acuity improves after treatment.
- There is no difference in acuity after treatment.
- There acuity or vision quality is worse after treatment.

The patient also needs to be reminded about the risks of surgery. These are less than before as a new flap does not need to be cut, but there is still a risk of scarring, haze and infection. Short-term symptoms that the patient may have had before could also re-occur such as starburst, haloes and dry eye.

RETREATMENT PROCEDURE

The prescription will be verified on the day of treatment by the surgeon or an optometrist in the clinic.

As the LASIK flap can be lifted for a considerable period after the initial treatment, creating another flap is not usually necessary. Under normal slit lamp illumination, the edge of the previous flap is located accurately. Once the surgeon has identified the flap edge, it is slightly raised using a Sinskey hook or a needle. There is more than one method of lifting the flap but it is not peeled back until the patient is on the laser bed. Once the flap has been lifted, the treatment is the same as with the original treatment.

Retreatment results and recovery

The patient's recovery is usually very similar to that of the initial treatment, although there is risk of epithelial ingrowth with relifting the flap. The vision tends to be very good after retreatment even though the risk of over or undercorrection is the same as with the initial treatment. For example, if the original treatment undercorrects a −8.00 DS eye by 10%, then the residual prescription will be 0.8 DS. This is very noticeable to the average myope. On retreatment, even if the undercorrection is still 10%, the residual myopia is only 0.08 DS, which is clinically insignificant. The vision is unlikely to regress significantly as the attempted treatment is usually small.

DISCHARGE

Between 3 and 6 months after treatment, the patient is usually ready to be discharged. A letter discharging the patient from the care of the clinic should be sent to the patient's general practitioner informing them of the successful outcome of treatment. The patient should also be advised to continue to have routine eye examinations on a regular basis even though they may not require spectacles or contact lenses. A discharge letter should also be sent to the patient's optometrist to ensure that the continued care of their eyes is not compromised by the lack of information.

Report to the optometrist

When writing the optometrist's report, it is good practice to include any information that might be useful in the future ocular management of the patient.

Pre-operative refractive error This is important as high myopes can have ocular features that are different (*e.g.* myopic crescents, peripheral retinal thinning). If features like these are noticed by a clinician who is unaware of the previous history of myopia, they could be interpreted as suspicious. Highly myopic eyes are also more susceptible to peripheral retinal degeneration and detachment. Refractive surgery does not alter this risk and it is important that these patients are still monitored routinely.

Postoperative refractive error If the patient notices a change in their vision, the examining optometrist will need to know if any residual prescription was present on discharge. In some cases, it can be difficult to differentiate between regression of a treatment and the natural progression of a patient's refractive error. Where the refractive error appears to change by fairly large amounts over a short period of time, it is certainly more suspicious and, in the absence of other clinical signs, referral back to the treating clinic may be indicated to monitor the regression in refractive error.

Corneal signs The postoperative cornea can look quite different to a normal 'untouched' cornea. There can be surgical debris, scarring at the edge of the flap or even microstriae present. All these things are normal after treatment, but in a non-treated eye, these signs would warrant referral for further investigation. It would be advisable to include information of any corneal signs present on discharge so that if other ocular signs manifest themselves, they are not interpreted as post-surgical signs.

Intraocular pressure The cornea can be significantly thinner after corneal refractive surgery and, as a result, the intraocular pressure appears lower even though it is actually the same. The Imbert-Fick Law upon which applanation tonometry is based states that the external force (W) against a sphere is equal to the pressure inside the sphere (P_I) multiplied by the area (A) that is applanated by the external force.

The prerequisites for this law do not apply to the eye. That is, the eye is not a perfect sphere bound by an infinitely thin, dry and flexible membrane. The Goldman applanation tonometer is calibrated to a 'normal' eye where the cornea is approximately 520–530 μm. Therefore, it follows that any change to corneal curvature, corneal thickness or ocular rigidity can alter the accuracy of an applanation tonometer. The change in readings cannot be simply equated to the degree of refractive change and so it is important that the IOP is recorded before and after treatment. This information needs to be forwarded on to the optometrist as it is important in the screening for glaucoma and potential management of IOP.

For example, a patient presents for a routine eye examination 2 years after refractive surgery. The IOP reading at this time was 23 mmHg. The optometrist has the records from the last eye examination and there appears to be no change in IOP so no action is taken. However, if the optometrist had received a report from the treating clinic that the patient's IOP measurement had dropped to 16 mmHg after treatment, the increase of 7 mmHg would have been noticed immediately. If the patient had not had treatment and the corneal thickness remained the same as before, the IOP reading would have been 30 mmHg. This alters the management of the patient considerably.

Pachymetry   Pre-operative corneal thickness measurements should also be included in any final report as it may aid the early diagnosis of glaucoma.

Other considerations

Keratometry readings   Keratometry is used prior to cataract extraction to calculate the power of the replacement intraocular lens (IOL). Inaccuracies arise in the IOL calculations as the instruments used to measure the corneal parameters are not designed for the post-refractive surgery cornea. Refractive surprise can be prevented in the future by forwarding on the pre-operative information[9] to the patient's general practitioner so that it can passed on to the relevant ophthalmologist should the need arise.

Topography images   Only the central corneal curvature is altered after LASIK, so the keratometry readings after treatment do not give an accurate impression of the corneal profile. Keratometry only measures the cornea at 4 points within the central 3–4 mm, but topography is able to measure the whole corneal surface at up to 11 000 points. This is useful if the patient is discharged but still needs contact lenses to correct their vision to an acceptable level. In cases where the ablation is decentred or if irregular astigmatism is present, the topography images will provide valuable information for selecting suitable lens parameters.

Before sending any reports to the patient's optometrist or general practitioner, it is important to ensure that the patient has consented for the information to be so used. In most cases, consent is obtained at the consultation stage or when the patient signs a consent form for surgery. Sample reports are given in Chart 9.1 and Chart 9.2. Printable versions are available from <www.optometryonline.net>.

Report to General Medical Practitioner

Practice/Clinic Name
Address
Telephone Nos

Date:

Re: Px Name:
       Px Address:

DOB:

The above patient has had LASIK treatment and is now being discharged from our care. We have recommended that the patient continues to have routine eye examinations with their own optometrist on a regular basis. The following information is for reference only and may be useful if the patient is referred to an ophthalmologist for further investigation in the future.

Date of treatment:

Date of further treatment (if applicable):

Pre-operative Refraction			**BCVA**
R:	/	/	6/
L:	/	/	6/

Postoperative Refraction			**BCVA**	**NVA**
R:	/	/	6/	N
L:	/	/	6/	N

Other measurements:

Pre-operative Intraocular Pressure	**Postoperative Intraocular Pressure**
R: (mmHg)	R: (mmHg)
L:	L:

Taken at: am/pm	Taken at: am/pm
Instrument used:	Instrument used:

Pre-operative Pachymetry	**Pre-operative Keratometry**	
R: μm	R: D @	D @
L: μm	L: D @	D @

Other information:

If you require further details, please do not hesitate to contact the clinic.

Yours faithfully,

Optometrist

Chart 9.1   Discharge report to general medical practitioner

Report to Optometrist

Practice/Clinic Name
Address
Telephone Nos

Date:

Re: Px Name:
     Px Address:

DOB:

The above patient has had LASIK treatment and is now being discharged from our care. We recommend that the patient has a routine eye examination within 12 months of discharge and after that, at your recommendation.

Date of treatment:

Date of futher treatment (if applicable):

Pre-operative Refraction   BCVA
R: /   /   6/
L: /   /   6/

Postoperative Unaided Acuity
R: 6/   N
L: 6/   N

Postoperative Refraction   BCVA   Near Add   NVA
R: /   /   6/   N
L: /   /   6/   N

Pre-operative Intraocular Pressure   Postoperative Intraocular Pressure
R: (mmHg)   R: (mmHg)
L: L:

Taken at: am/pm   Taken at: am/pm
Instrument used: Instrument used:

Pre-operative Pachymetry   Pre-operative Keratometry
R: μm   R: D @   D @
L: μm   L: D @   D @

Other information:

Please note that this is not a prescription for spectacles. If you require further details, please do not hesitate to contact the clinic.

Yours faithfully,

Optometrist

Chart 9.2 Discharge report to optometrist

The Royal College of Ophthalmologists' standards for laser refractive surgery state that a copy of the following be given to the patient:
Pre-operative keratometry
Pre-operative pachymetry
Pre- and postoperative best corrected acuity
Pre- and postoperative intraocular pressure
Pre-operative and stabilised postoperative refraction

ISSUING A PRESCRIPTION FOR SPECTACLES

There may be some instances where the patient may wish to acquire spectacles after discharge:

- Presbyope needs reading spectacles or varifocals.
- Patient with monovision needs prescription for reading small print.
- Patient with monovision needs prescription for driving at night.
- Patient with residual myopia where full treatment was not possible.

It should be explained to the patients that a prescription is not merely a refraction measurement, but a clinical decision based upon the results of several assessments such as binocular vision assessment and visual task analysis. As the patient is now discharged, the optometrist needs to consider the *Sight Testing (examination and prescription) (No 2) Regulations 1989*.[10] If issuing a prescription, it is advisable to carry out a full eye examination rather than just refraction, or to refer the patient back to their own optometrist.

References

1. Benitez-del-Castillo JM, del Rio T, Iradier T *et al.* Decrease in tear secretion and corneal sensitivity after laser *in situ* keratomileusis. Cornea 2001;20:30–32.
2. Asano-Kato N, Toda I, Hori-Komai Y *et al.* Epithelial ingrowth after laser *in situ* keratomileusis: clinical features and possible mechanisms. Am J Ophthalmol 2002;134:801–807.
3. Ivarsen A, Laurberg T, Moller-Pedersen T. Characterisation of corneal fibrotic wound repair at the LASIK flap margin. Br J Ophthalmol 2003;87:1272–1278.
4. BJ, Kowal L. Diplopia after refractive surgery: occurrence and prevention. Arch Ophthalmol 2003;121:315–321.
5. Miranda D, Smith SD, Krueger RR. Comparison of flap thickness reproducibility using microkeratomes with a second motor for advancement. Ophthalmology 2003;110:1931–1934.
6. Spadea L, Palmieri G, Mosca L *et al.* Iatrogenic keratectasia following laser *in situ* keratomileusis. J Refract Surg 2002;18:475–480.

7. Giledi O, Daya SM. Unexpected flap thickness in laser *in situ* keratomileusis. J Cataract Refract Surg 2003;29:1825–1826.

8. Cua IY, Pepose JS. Proper positioning of the plume evacuator in the VISX Star3 excimer laser minimizes central island formation in patients undergoing laser *in situ* keratomileusis. J Refract Surg 2003;19:309–315.

9. Feiz V, Mannis MJ, Garcia-Ferrer FV. Intraocular lens power calculation after laser *in situ* keratomileusis for myopia and hyperopia: a standardized approach. Cornea 2001;20:792–797.

10. The Sight Testing (Examination and prescription) (No 2) Regulations 1989.

Chapter **10**

The future: will LASEK supersede LASIK?

OVERVIEW

LASIK and PRK are tried, tested and audited techniques that have been successful in treating ammetropia. Surgeons are constantly looking to improve the surgical techniques and procedures that they carry out. As the collective experience of these surgeons increases, new variations of procedures or techniques are evolving. This chapter will look as the relatively new procedure of LASEK and discuss the advantages and disadvantages when compared to LASIK.

CONTENTS

INTRODUCTION

Although LASEK has a similar name to LASIK it is in fact a modified form of PRK. It is a relatively new method of treatment that was first reported in the ophthalmic literature around 1999. Massimo Camellin devised the acronym LASEK but in fact, the technique was first described by Kenneth Hoffer in 1990 although called by a different name.[1] It reduces some of the risks of PRK such as haze and regression and those associated with flap creation in LASIK.[2]

Prior to LASIK, laser refractive surgery was not seen as an option for many patients as the risks associated with PRK did not appear to outweigh the potential benefits. There is also the inconvenience factor. PRK was rarely done as a bilateral treatment and the visual recovery could take several days. Having to take a few days of work to have PRK, and then to need more time off to have the second eye treated was too disruptive for many. Patients may also have been put off by the probability of ocular pain as the cornea re-epithelialised.

LASIK on the other hand is able to deliver bilateral treatments with very little discomfort and rapid visual recovery. Patients are able to have treatment with minimum disruption to their busy lives and, although there are risks, these do not negate the convenience of a quick procedure with reliable outcomes. However, not all patients are able to have LASIK or may be at a higher risk of having flap complications. LASEK may be a possible solution for these patients.

LASEK CANDIDATES

The prescription range that a surgeon will treat can vary. The risk of haze and regression that was associated with higher myopic PRK treatments prescriptions is less with LASEK.[3] Some surgeons are still opting for a more conservative approach and will only treat up to 3 or 4 dioptres of myopia. Those patients that have insufficient cornea to leave a 250 µm stromal bed after the LASIK flap has been cut may be suitable LASEK candidates. LASEK may also be more suitable for patients that are at high risk of microkeratome related complications. Patients that are already diagnosed with dry eye may be more suitable for LASEK as there is a reduced risk of dry eye problems postoperatively.

LASEK vs PRK vs LASIK

LASEK and PRK procedures are also known as surface ablation treatments and involve removing the epithelium and then treating the stroma underneath. With PRK, the epithelium is completely removed and must then regenerate. The patient will feel mild to moderately severe pain during the first 72 hours after treatment. With LASEK, the epithelium is folded or rolled back and then replaced after the treatment. Covering the epithelial wound with an epithelial flap immediately after treatment may reduce pain.[2] Although alcohol is toxic to the epithelium, some cells remain viable.[4] This may reduce the epithelial trigger which induces haze formation.[5] In the LASIK procedure, the flap is cut by a microkeratome in the anterior stroma and excimer laser is applied to the deeper stroma. Bowman's membrane is retained. The LASEK flap is epithelial only and is created by delaminating the basement membrane. The laser treatment is then carried out on the anterior stromal surface and Bowman's membrane is ablated away over the treatment area. Details of the LASEK treatment can be seen below.

LASEK – THE PROCEDURE

- The cornea is anaesthetised using a topical agent. The eye that is not being treated may be covered with an eye pad.
- The eye area is prepared and the eyelashes draped. The patient is asked to look at the fixation target.
- The speculum is inserted.
- A trephine is a circular cutting device with a flattened section usually placed at 12 o'clock to create a hinge. This is pushed downwards and with a twisting motion to create an epithelial incision 80 μm deep which forms the flap edge.
- An alcohol chamber of is placed centrally onto the cornea and is filled with a 20% alcohol.
- After 20–30 seconds (or longer in some cases), the surgeon uses a sponge to soak up the alcohol.
- The cornea is then irrigated to remove any residual alcohol.
- The flap edges are then lifted along the trephine mark using a purpose designed instrument and the epithelium is then peeled back with corneal flap elevator.
- The exposed Bowmann's membrane is then checked for residual epithelium.
- The laser ablation takes place.
- The epithelium is gently replaced.
- A bandage contact is then inserted.

RISKS AND COMPLICATIONS

Surgical complications

Possible laser complications such as decentred ablation and central islands are low as with LASIK. The main surgical complication associated with LASEK is of flap loss. If this occurs, then the procedure proceeds as for PRK. The adherence of the epithelial cells to the basement membrane varies between individuals and in some cases prolonged alcohol exposure is required to create a separation. Alcohol is toxic to the epithelium and the amount of cell death is dependent on alcohol concentration and exposure duration.[4] Some surgeons think this may cause an increase in the pain felt by the patient postoperatively.

Short-term postoperative risk/complications

- There is a risk of infection postoperatively as the epithelium regenerates. This is minimised with the use of a topical antibiotic prophylactically.

- Abrasion or poor epithelial adhesion in some patients may result in slower recovery and increased discomfort postoperatively.

- In the case of flap loss or if a viable flap cannot be created during treatment, the patient feel moderate-to-severe pain postoperatively which may be controlled with oral and topical analgesics.

- Most patients experience a mild degree of haze postoperatively which may cause a reduction of vision and haloes around lights. Significant haze is managed with the use of topical anti-inflammatory or anti-metabolite agents where necessary (see box on Mitomycin C).

- There is a risk of dry eye postoperatively.

> *Mitomycin C*
> Haze formation after surface treatments has been the focus of many studies and the use of the powerful antimetabolite Mitomycin C immediately after ablation is known to inhibit this response.[6,7] Mitomycin C is a cytotoxic agent which inhibits DNA synthesis and is effective at preventing cell division. This reduces the healing response and the formation of scar tissue. The protocols for using this controversial agent in refractive surgery vary between surgeons. Most surgeons will only use Mitomycin C prophylactically on high myopic treatments or to treat existing haze. When used, it is usually used in a concentration of 0.02% or 0.03% for 15–45 seconds, then copiously irrigated off. The use of this DNA inhibiting agent is controversial as the long-term effects on the cornea are not fully known.

Long-term complications

- There is a risk of under or overcorrection by the laser. This may mean a difference in the prescription and acuity between the eyes.

- Persistent haze can cause scarring and the loss of up to 2 lines of best corrected acuity is possible (BVCA). However haze of greater than grade 1 is unusual[3,5] and grade 1 or less is unlikely to affect BCVA.

- A persistent epithelial defect may occur and can cause pain and watering of the eye as well as increasing the risk of infection. If this persists, a reduction or aberrations in the vision may occur.

- Regression of the laser treatment can occur with time and the patient may require further treatment.

Other side effects

Due to the changed shape of the cornea it may be more difficult to wear contact lenses postoperatively.

TYPICAL POSTOPERATIVE SYMPTOMS

Although the procedure itself is painless due to the anaesthesia, the patient will feel some discomfort when the anaesthetic wears off. Some patients may experience severe discomfort while the epithelium heals; if there is significant pain, analgesics can be used. The discomfort will be significantly better after 48 hours. A protective pad or shield may be placed over the eye for the first 24 hours.

By day 3 or 4 the patient will feel comfortable and the vision will feel less blurred. Patients are advised not to drive until after they have had their vision checked and it has been confirmed to be adequate.

Postoperative care

This will vary from surgeon to surgeon, but the first aftercare is usually carried out within the first 4 days after treatment. Some surgeons prefer to see the patient daily until the contact lens is removed. This is usually done on day 4 and, depending upon the status of the epithelium, the surgeon may choose to insert a new bandage lens if necessary. The visual acuity is checked, but the patient is not expected to achieve the target unaided acuity until 1 week after treatment. The cornea will be checked for any early signs of haze. It is common practice for surgeons to prescribe topical anti-inflammatory agents prophylactically for short-term use to minimise the risk of haze formation.

The patient is then checked after one week when a reliable refraction is more likely to be obtained. By this stage, the cornea should be completely re-epithelialised with no sign of an epithelial defect.[8,9] The practitioner should also look for soft lens related infiltrates (Figure 10.1) as the bandage lens is worn continuously for up to 4 days postoperatively. There may also be a build up of

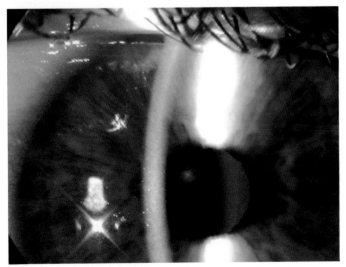

Figure 10.1 Soft contact lens related infiltrate

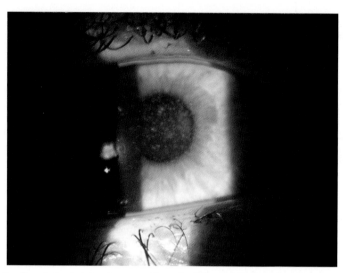

Figure 10.2   Punctate staining is seen after a toxicity reaction

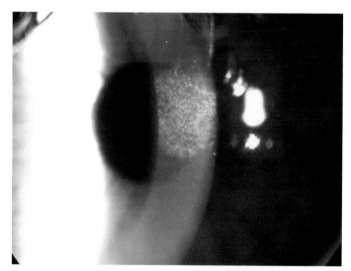

Figure 10.3   Corneal haze may be seen after LASEK or PRK

preservative in the lens if multidose topical agents have been used which could cause a toxicity reaction (Figure 10.2).

At 1 month, the vision and refractive error are generally stable. Mild haze may be seen, though it is rarely greater than grade 1.[3,5] If PRK was performed due to the loss of the epithelial flap, then the risk of haze is greater and is usually maximal at 1–3 months' postoperatively.[10] If significant haze is seen (Figure 10.3), referral to the surgeon is required as treatment may be required.

By 6 months, the eye there should be no significant haze and the vision should be stable. A further check at 12 months is advisable to ensure that the patient has achieved a stable refraction and that risk of late onset haze has passed. This has not been documented with LASEK yet but is a known risk of PRK.[9] The patient can be discharged if the refraction is stable and the patient is happy.

DISCUSSION

LASEK appears to have few risks and the procedure is less invasive than LASIK; however, it is not the first choice procedure for most surgeons. The reasons for this are multifactorial.

Patient recommendation

It is a relatively new procedure and does not yet have the same reputation as LASIK among patients, so is in less demand. The recovery period when compared to LASIK is slower and so does not create the same 'wow' factor which motivates personal recommendation from treated patient to prospective patient.

FDA approval

In the US, the Food and Drug Administration (FDA) approves drugs and devices for medical procedures, but not the actual procedures themselves. Currently, the use of the excimer laser for LASEK is not FDA-approved. However, those lasers that have earned approval based on PRK or LASIK data can be used in LASEK procedures. The use of approved devices in such an instance is called an 'off-label' use. As the approved lasers have proven safe and effective in other procedures, ophthalmologists may use them off-label if they feel it is in their patients' best interest to do so. As the use of excimer lasers in LASEK is not FDA approved, advertising of the procedure is restricted. This may have an impact on the confidence and awareness of the procedure among patients.

Haze and discomfort

Advocates of LASEK claim that postoperative discomfort and haze formation is less than with PRK and that visual recovery is better. Despite studies showing excellent visual results,[3,5] there is a belief among some surgeons that LASEK is a re-packaged PRK and that the decrease in haze and regression is more due to improved lasers and drug regimens than the technique itself.[10,11] Haze formation may also be linked to the surgeon's technique for creating the epithelial flap as it is not straightforward and there is a learning curve.[7] The benefits of the epithelial flap still need to be validated as there are studies which do not show any significant difference between PRK and LASEK.[8,9]

Future developments

Flap creation in LASIK has been shown in some studies to increase higher order aberrations.[15,16] Wavefront-guided ablations that are based upon the untreated eye result in the correction of aberrations that were detected prior to the flap being cut only. This limits the benefits of wavefront technology. The use of wave-front-guided treatment with surface ablation may remove this limitation as the cornea re-epithelialises after LASEK/PRK and flap-related aberrations are not induced. This theory needs more research as one study found no significant difference in the visual performance of eyes that had undergone PRK when compared to LASIK.[17]

CONCLUSION

The creation of the LASEK flap can be done in several ways with variations in the shape of the flap, the type and strength of alcohol used, the duration of alcohol exposure and the way the flap is lifted. Until the procedure is standardised, it may be difficult to get consistent findings for this procedure. The postoperative recovery period may be reduced in LASEK if a less traumatic method of creating the epithelial flap was developed. However, the convenience that LASIK offers in terms of rapid visual recovery and minimal pain is hard to beat, and until LASEK can do that it will not seriously threaten the popularity of LASIK.

References

1. Hoffer K. Reflections on the origins of LASEK, 1990. Rev Ophthalmol 2003;11:10/05.
2. Camellin M. Laser epithelial keratomileusis for myopia. J Refract Surg 2003;19:666–670.
3. Bilgihan K, Hondur A, Hasanreisoglu B. Laser subepithelial keratomileusis for myopia of −6 to −10 diopters with astigmatism with the MEL60 laser. J Refract Surg 2004;20:121–126.
4. Chen CC, Chang JH, Lee JB et al. Human corneal epithelial cell viability and morphology after dilute alcohol exposure. Invest Ophthalmol Vis Sci 2002;43:2593–2602.
5. Gabler B, Winkler von Mohrenfels C, Herrmann et al. Laser epithelial keratomileusis (LASEK) for treatment of myopia up to −6.0 D. Results from 108 eyes after 12 months. Ophthalmologe 2004;101:146–152.
6. Carones F, Vigo L, Scandola E et al. Evaluation of the prophylactic use of mitomycin-C to inhibit haze formation after photorefractive keratectomy. J Cataract Refract Surg 2002;28:2088–2095.
7. Xu H, Liu S, Xia X, Huang P et al. Mitomycin C reduces haze formation in rabbits after excimer laser photorefractive keratectomy. J Refract Surg 2001;17:342–349.
8. Litwak S, Zadok D, Garcia-de Quevedo V et al. Laser-assisted subepithelial keratectomy versus photorefractive keratectomy for the correction of myopia. A prospective comparative study. J Cataract Refract Surg 2002;28:1330–1333.
9. Pirouzian A, Thornton JA, Ngo S. A randomized prospective clinical trial comparing laser subepithelial keratomileusis and photorefractive keratectomy. Ophthalmology 2004;122:11–16.
10. Lohmann CP, Gartry DS, Muir MK, Timberlake GT, Fitzke FW, Marshall J. Corneal haze after excimer laser refractive surgery: objective measurements and functional implications. Eur J Ophthalmol 1991;1:173–180.

11. Kuo IC, Lee SM, Hwang DG. Late-onset corneal haze and myopic regression after photorefractive keratectomy (PRK). Cornea 2004;23:350–355.
12. Bethke W. LASEK: where does it fit in? Rev Ophthalmol 2002;09/07.
13. Bruce Jackson W. When complications come to the surface. Rev Ophthalmol 2002;09/07.
14. Chalita MR, Tekwani NH, Krueger RR. Laser epithelial keratomileusis: outcome of initial cases performed by an experienced surgeon. J Refract Surg 2003;19:412–415.
15. Porter J, MacRae S, Yoon G, Roberts C, Cox IG, Williams DR. Separate effects of the microkeratome incision and laser ablation on the eye's wave aberration. Am J Ophthalmol 2003;136:327–337.
16. Pallikaris IG, Kymionis GD, Panagopoulou SI et al. Induced optical aberrations following formation of a laser in situ keratomileusis flap. J Cataract Refract Surg 2002;28:1737–1741.
17. Ninomiya S, Maeda N, Kuroda T et al. Comparison of ocular higher-order aberrations and visual performance between photorefractive keratectomy and laser in situ keratomileusis for myopia. Semin Ophthalmol 2003;18:29–34.

Index

Note: page numbers in *italic* type refer to tables and in **bold** type to figures.